An Epidemiological Odyssey

Dr. George Pollock

An Epidemiological Odyssey

The Evolution of Communicable Disease Control

Springer

Dr. George Pollock
Honorary Senior Research Fellow
Department of Public Health and Epidemiology
University of Birmingham
Edgbaston
Birmingham B15 2TT
United Kingdom

ISBN 978-94-017-8328-6 ISBN 978-94-007-3998-7 (eBook)
DOI 10.1007/978-94-007-3998-7
Springer Dordrecht Heidelberg New York London

Softcover reprint of the hardcover 1st edition 2012

Printed on acid-free paper

Springer is part of Springer Science+Business Media (www.springer.com)

"To Edie Kate Pollock, whose odyssey is just beginning."

Foreword

Epidemics of communicable diseases are a natural occurrence co-existing with life itself. They have been reported in literature from the Bible onwards including references with comment in the plays of William Shakespeare. In early times they were generally referred to as plagues. The invention of the microscope led to their cause being identified in transmission of micro-organisms by humans or other animals. Protection from disease by quarantine of infected persons was followed by vaccination. With the introduction of antibiotic therapy there became a belief in the mid-twentieth century that communicable disease could be eliminated from the planet. This proved to be true for smallpox and possibly for poliomyelitis by programmes of vaccination, but otherwise this soon became apparent as a politician's dream. Resistance to antibiotics by organisms, emergence of new micro-organisms, particularly the human immunodeficiency virus (HIV) and increased of travel soon put an end to such beliefs. It therefore becomes essential that people at large understand how such beliefs came about and how epidemics can occur in order that they may be avoided in the future. That is the purpose of this treatise by Dr. George Pollock. A critical analysis of the history of epidemics, is followed by reports of personal experiences. These are related as sufferer, observer, National Health Service consultant and now historian. There are few who can have had the opportunity to describe at first hand how the risks and actual occurrence of epidemics affect both the individual patient and the community. He experienced the initial appearance of potential epidemics, and relates the measures taken to combat their spread. The reaction of those advising government is reported, giving a lively insight to the processes of management under stress as well as the reactions of the populace and its handling by the media in a number of specific instances are described for posterity. The past successes and failures to combat communicable diseases are set down as personal experiences for posterity. The misjudgement of politicians in 1974 of dismantling the organisations for control of communicable diseases that had been developed over the previous half century is emphasised. The measures taken to reintroduce systems of control of infection particularly surveillance at local, district, national and European level are detailed The importance of considering the effects of an epidemic on social, mystical and religious thought must be appreciated. This book is both an autobiography and an historical report including finally a perspective from today with hopes for the future. The book is therefore essential reading for those who wish to prevent overwhelming epidemics in any part of the world especially if they intend to propose changes in health care structure.

Professor Keith Shinton
Emeritus Professor of Postgraduate Medical Education
University of Warwick
United Kingdom

Preface

This book had its origin in a "valedictory" presentation which I gave at Birmingham University in December 2008 to mark the end of my honorary senior lectureship. The fact that the earlier part of the book constitutes a reworking of familiar historical narrative represents a kind of paradox for me as I grew up in a household where Henry Ford's dictum that "History is bunk" was the received wisdom, the result of my father's having worked at the Ford Motor Company in Detroit in the late 1920s.

My conversion came much later as the result of taking my young son to see the film Richard III, in which the combination of Shakespeare's dialogue, Olivier's acting and Walton's music had the power to present historical events as a gripping drama. By a curious coincidence, at about the same time, I came across an account of the disease known as the "English sweat" and reflected that, had Henry's victorious troops known what was about to assail them shortly after Bosworth Field, they would perhaps been less triumphalist.

I have not attempted to create a continuous narrative in the first three chapters, rather a series of epidemiological snapshots of England at times of significance, such as the rapid assembly of a network of local public health authorities when cholera breached the supposedly protective wall of maritime quarantine. From Chap. 4 onwards I have tried to present the account from a personal point of view, as an individual sometimes on the periphery of events, frequently affected by organisational change but only rarely in a position to influence it. In doing so, I hope to have been able to re-create the atmosphere of a number of situations: the chattering teeth of a line-up of shivering 10-year olds nervously awaiting their first inoculation; the surreal absurdity of an emergency 1-day promotion to ensure that both Army Regulations and WHO requirements were met; the horror of learning, many years afterwards, that my determination to prevent a smallpox outbreak had led to my unwittingly breaking, probably, several laws. Understandably, I hope, my adopted home town of Coventry receives many mentions, as I have spent the greater part of my professional life in that vibrant city.

I had originally intended that the continuous thread running through the book should be a plea for communicable diseases to be taken seriously, even in a Developed country like England, in a world where no one is further than 72 h away from any source of infection. However I could not really prevent the account from developing, in parts, into a kind of autobiography; I hope that the reader will excuse this.

George Pollock

Acknowledgements

My debts in the preparation of this book lie principally in a number of libraries. I must first thank Professor Sir Liam Donaldson, at the time Chief Medical Officer of the Department of Health in London, for allowing me to have access to the Department's Information Services unit in Leeds, and also Natalie Dudgeon, Senior Librarian and her staff at that location for their untiring assistance. I am also extremely grateful to Shona McLean and her staff at the Wellcome Unit for the History of Medicine in Oxford for their considerable help over a wide range of topics. I owe a great deal to Sheila Adams and her colleagues at the Coventry History Centre for making available to me the extremely valuable archive material which allowed me to give much of the book a local focus. Finally I must express particular thanks to the staff at Birmingham University Library who kindly granted me long-term loans on over 20 of their textbooks.

Two individuals deserve special mention. Margaret Pelling, Reader in the Social History Medicine at Oxford, gave me wise advice on getting the balance of the book right, and Philip Mortimer, Consultant Microbiologist at the Health Protection Agency, was able to provide me with fascinating insights into the development of the Public Health Laboratory Service.

George Pollock

Contents

Chapter 1
Early Concepts of Communicability

I first came across the concept that a disease could be infectious when I was about 5 years old and had a bad cold. My mother told me that someone had "*given me the smit*." From her explanation I formed the idea that "*the smit*" was like a tiny blob of jelly that one child could give to another, rather like a small sweet, and I protested that I could not remember receiving any such gift.

Thirty years later, when I was on a Council of Europe Fellowship attached to the City Health Department in Amsterdam, and learning Dutch in the process, I discovered that their word for infectious was *be**smet**telijk* and I realised that my mother's Aberdeen dialect word had European connections. (I subsequently found that many colloquial expressions from my hometown had their roots in Dutch and the Scandinavian languages, the result of the city being both a busy fishing and mercantile port. I was particularly exposed to such influences as my maternal grandfather was a North Sea trawl fisherman.)

How far back can one go in endeavouring to find a reasonable starting point in this quest? According to Cockburn (1977) to the origins of life itself, when cells, including bacteria, and viruses were formed? In which case one has also to consider the impact of subsequent evolution of mammals, including primates, and the parasitic relationships which the microbiological world has developed with these later species. Although this study is primarily concerned with human disease transmission, it clearly cannot exclude infections transmitted from both domesticated and wild animals to humans as all three have lived in relatively close contact since earliest times.

Additionally one must consider the whole concept of what we understand by communities which on a macro scale developed when movements of the earth's crust created the continents as we now know them, but which at the other end of the scale evolved when nomadic hunting-gathering declined in favour of people settling down in a locality to grow their own grain and husband their domestic animals. Cunliffe (1983) has described how, during the course of the late fifth millennium BC, settlers from the European continent came to Britain with their seed corn and domesticated livestock so that within 1,000 years or so, a settled way of farming life

G. Pollock, *An Epidemiological Odyssey: The Evolution of Communicable Disease Control*, DOI 10.1007/978-94-007-3998-7_1,

had spread throughout the British Isles, with people now tied to the land and local communities growing in size. Cockburn (1977) has clearly illustrated the epidemiological impact of these changes in terms of man's acquisition of pathogens from not only cattle, pigs and sheep but also fowl, ducks and geese. He also suggests that there was always a great deal of scope for cross-infection between man and wild animals e.g. because of people defecating in their fields whose crops might later be raided by creatures such as monkeys.

The size and stability of the local population group would clearly have always been important factors. Acquired infections would stay within that local community until an infected person moved to another locality, thereby creating a potential source of infection elsewhere. An account of how such small primitive communities developed into the earliest civilisations, now clearly shown by archeological evidence to have been settled societies with forms of government, legal systems and shared cultures is beyond the scope of this work, nor would it be likely to contribute much to the central theme. Accordingly these established ancient civilisations will be regarded as the natural starting point in this search, especially those which grew up on major rivers such as the Indus, Tigris, Euphrates and Nile.

An issue of major significance which needs to be introduced at this point is the apparently overwhelming influence which supernatural beliefs have had, since earliest times, on man's thinking about life, health, disease and cures. Whether one refers to such beliefs as religion, spirituality, animism or magic (or, for that matter, pure nonsense), depends on one's personal and cultural viewpoint. The importance of the issue, from the point of view of this study, is that it seems that such beliefs have always existed in parallel with attempts to explain disease and cure in an empirical manner, by observation and interpretation from evidence, and on many occasions the former have inhibited or frustrated the latter. Cave drawings by primitive man represent perhaps the first illustrations of convictions of this kind, but every generation can be seen to subscribe, to a certain extent, to such beliefs, even the twenty-first century having so-called "alternative medicine" alongside "evidence-based medicine."

It is clear that many of the ancient civilisations, from the Mesopotamian, Egyptian and those of the Indus Valley onwards, set a considerable value on personal cleanliness, if only for a privileged elite, and this is generally believed to have been allied to spirituality and religious purity, although personal comfort could also very reasonably have been an objective. It is possible that such communities which had developed elaborate drainage systems, centuries ahead of their time, were *unwittingly* reducing the risk of intestinal infections, and the shaving of their heads and bodies by priests would certainly have contributed to the reduction of louse-borne diseases and other infestations. And so some elements of good public health practice may well have developed to some extent for reasons totally unconnected with health considerations.

There is also a great deal of evidence that infectious diseases existed in recognisable forms from earliest times. But this does not really indicate to what extent in those days people were aware that such diseases could be communicated from one person to another. Parts of The Old Testament, thought to have been written by

Moses between 1440 and 1400 BC, certainly gave clear instructions to priests concerning the measures to be taken to prevent the spread of leprosy, mainly isolating sufferers from the general community. However it was not until around 600 BC in India that an eminent surgeon called Sushruta gave a good clinical description in a Sanskrit text, *Sushruta Samhita*, how the disease, being contagious, could be carried from a sufferer to a healthy person (Buhier 1886).

It seems that Hippocrates of Cos (460–375 BC), the most prominent physician of the Classical Greek age, in his many essays on health and disease, used the term leprosy, along with others such as cholera and typhus, in only a rather imprecise manner which did not necessarily represent the clinical conditions which we understand by these terms nowadays. Hippocrates did, however, give detailed descriptions of a wide range of infectious diseases including pulmonary tuberculosis, mumps, poliomyelitis, meningitis, tonsillitis and malaria. He also clearly understood what one might refer to as the *pathology* of infection—the fever and swelling as part of the immune response; additionally he believed in the concept of contagion (Pappas et al. 2008). Sometimes, however, this latter factor seemed to be lacking in his descriptions. This seems surprising given that he has the reputation of being the first to apply a scientific approach to the observation of disease. For example in Hippocrates Epidemics Book 1 (circa 400 BC) he states "*All these fevers described attacked great numbers*" and also pointed out that "*These things occurred to those affected with the complaints described above, and then to many persons at first without them*," both statements which would tend to indicate transmission from person to person, although the account makes no mention of contagion as the cause of these phenomena. Perhaps his concept of contagion related more frequently to disease acquired from the environment, such as malaria from swampy areas and diarrhea from consuming certain waters or inadequately cooked food.

Both Hippocrates and his follower Galen of Pergamon (129–210 AD), a Greek physician who moved to Rome and became surgeon to the gladiators believed that epidemics could be caused by corrupt air, an imbalance of the bodily humours and adverse astrological positions. Galen went so far as to state that "…the nature of disease is to be found in man's temperament, the structure of his parts, his physiological and psychological dynamism…" (Nutton 1983). The Hippocratic writings were, of course, being put together against a background of civic concern for healthy cities in Greece. One example of this, according to Rosen (1958), was the practice from about 600 BC of municipal physicians being appointed on a salaried basis by the larger towns to advise on the health of the population and the prevention of epidemics.

Much earlier than Galen, a Roman scholar and gentleman farmer, Marcus Terentius Varro (116–27 BC), appears to have been the first to postulate the idea of communicability as we currently understand the term in the twenty-first century. In *De Re Rustica* Book I Chapter 12, written in 36 BC, he warned that precautions should be taken in the neighbourhood of swamps because "*crescunt animalia quaedam minuta, quae non possunt oculi consequi, et per aera intus in corpus per os ac nares perveniunt atque efficiunt difficilis morbos*," "there breed certain minute creatures which cannot be seen by the eyes but which by air enter the body through the mouth and nose and lead to serious diseases" (Pollock AF, 2009, Personal communication: email to author dated 11th March 2009). Hippocrates would probably have had no quarrel with this advice from an environmental point of view. [An interesting comment on the dangers of swamps was added by Vitruvius Pollio in *De Architectura*, written in the First Century AD, namely that when sea water was mixed with marshy soil the danger was less, and that towns located there might remain healthy (Nutton 1983).] There is, however, no evidence that this remarkable vision of the world of microbiology made any impact on Roman thinking about health and disease. Adler's (2004)view of this was that the Romans chose to "tough things out," in the manner of their courageous ancestors, rather than adopt a listening attitude to the doctrines of medicine. In fact, nearly 1,600 years had to pass before the idea reappeared, quite independently, in the writings of the Veronese physician Giralamo Fracastoro.

What *did* mark out the Roman approach to public health was the concept of an integrated system of aqueducts delivering fresh water for drinking and bathing, and sewers for disposing of human excrement which was carried away by the waste water from the baths and toilets. As in the case of the elaborate drainage systems in many of the ancient civilisations referred to above, these arrangements must have prevented a great deal of intestinal infection. In fact, in *De Aquis Urbis Romae*, Sextus Julius Frontinus. water commissioner for Rome from 97 to 104 AD, declared that "by his labors he had not only made Rome cleaner and its air purer, but had also removed the causes of disease which previously had given the city a bad reputation" (Rosen 1958). Such benefits clearly would have been felt throughout the Roman Empire including Britain.

On reflection it was clearly in Britain's best interests that the Romans had decided to invade and conquer the island although it was probably some time before the natives saw the situation in that light. As Churchill (1956) pointed out in his *History of the English-Speaking Peoples*, the Roman occupation meant that Britain, for a period of nearly 300 years, enjoyed the most comfortable times which its inhabitants had ever had. Towns, the essence of civilised life, had water supplies brought in by channels which followed the slope of the ground, public baths, lavatories and main drains, and the more wealthy citizens had central heating from a hypocaust, the raised floor-level beneath which warm air circulated. Earl (1983) has described how the remains of many of these features are still visible at Wroxeter, Shropshire, in its time the fourth largest Roman town in Britain. The fact that these facilities were initially brought into being essentially for the occupying armies or governing classes is irrelevant; the benefits in due course became available to many of the local inhabitants. The influence of the Christian religion in England was barely felt at this point but, as Earl (1983) has pointed out, some of the Roman soldiers and traders had brought their Christian beliefs with them, evidence for this including a fourth century mosaic representation of Christ from Hinton St Mary, Dorset, now in the British Museum. The later impact of Christianity on the subject of this work is described below.

When the Romans finally withdrew from Britain, as their Empire disintegrated around 410 AD, what happened for the next 200 years or so is very obscure. The period is frequently referred to as the beginning of the *Dark Ages*, an evocative and menacing but imprecise term, interpreted in a variety of ways but one which many reasonably regard as signifying an era with no reliable documents or records to indicate what was happening in Britain during that period. Presumably some of the Roman influences persisted for a period but there is some evidence that towns with their public health infrastructure decayed quite rapidly because of sheer neglect and these urban facilities were not renewed by the Barbarians, Jutes Angles and Saxons, who succeeded them. Porter (1999) describes the situation from the fifth century onwards as an awkward moulding together of the cultures of both the Roman heritage and the Barbarian invaders, alongside the teachings of Christian religion.

It was not until 731, the year in which Bede, a monk in the Northumbrian monastery at Jarrow, completed his *Ecclesiastical History of the English People* was there any reliable record of English society at that time. Although the book focused essentially on the work of the Church, Bede took the opportunity of commenting on its attitude towards the social beliefs and practices of the era. The culture of maintaining health by exercise, sensible diet and avoiding hazardous environments etc., Hippocratic traditions brought to England by the Romans, was replaced by the Christian doctrine of disease being the result of human sinning (presumed to be universal!) so that cure or recovery could come about only by prayer. Accordingly natural explanations of health and disease had to give way to belief in supernatural healing. For example, in Book IV, Chapter X, translated by J Stevens (1723) and revised by JA Giles (1847), Bede writes about a blind woman who has her sight restored:

> *There lived in that neighbourhood a certain earl, whose wife was seized with a dimness in her eyes, which at length became so bad, that she could not see the least glimpse of light: having continued some time in total darkness, on a sudden she bethought herself that she might recover her lost sight, if she were carried to the monastery of the nuns, and there pray for the same, at the relics of the saints.........and having long prayed there on her knees, she did not fail to be heard, for as she rose from prayer, before she went out of the place, she received the gift of sight which she had desired; and whereas she had been led there by her servants, she now returned home joyfully without help.*

Further on, in Book IV, Chapter XXXI, Bede describes how a man is cured of palsy:

> *This man........was returning home, when on a sudden, about half way, he was seized with a sudden distemper in his body, insomuch that he fell down, and having lain some time, he could scarcely rise again. When at last he got up, he felt one half of his body, from the head to the foot, struck with palsy, and with much difficulty got home with the help of a staff..........In this weak condition, a good thought came into his mind, which was to go to the church, the best way he could, to the tomb of the reverend father Cuthbert, and there, on his knees, and there beg of the Divine Goodness to be delivered from that disease............In the midst of his prayers, he fell as it were into a stupor...........He then awoke and rose up in perfect health.*

An interesting point is made by Willan (1821) to the effect that the official conversion of England to the Christian religion in 597 led to greater contact with the peoples of Italy, France and Belgium so that "epidemical and contagious disease prevailing on the continent at the close of the sixth century would necessarily be communicated to the English kingdoms." Bede, himself, in Book III, Chapter XXVII, describes an event which gives support to this notion:

> *In the same year of our Lord 664 an eclipse of the sun occurred about ten o'clock in the morning on the third of May, and a sudden plague which first decimated the southern parts of Britain, and later spread into Northumbria, brought widespread death to its people.*

And in Book IV, Chapter XXX, Bede draws attention to the importance of the Christian Faith to protect against this plague:

> *While the plague caused a heavy death-toll in the province, Sighere and his people abandoned the mysteries of the Christian Faith, and relapsed into paganism. For the king himself. together with many of the nobles and common folk, loved this life and sought no other, having no belief in a future life. But Sebbi his fellow king and colleague held loyally to the Faith which he and his people had accepted, and, as will appear later, remained faithful and ended his days happily.*

Although the Church's teaching—emphasising supernatural healing—clearly brushed aside a great deal of the legacy of what had been brought to England in terms of scientific thought, it has to be accepted that the clergy were, in fact, the only educated people remaining. Additionally it was only in the monasteries that such rudiments of public health infrastructure as water supplies and sewage disposal continued to exist; this taken in conjunction with the religious orthodoxy that cleanliness was next to Godliness did impose a sort of elementary practice of hygiene.

Commenting on this "sudden plague" of 664, referred to by Bede, Creighton (1894) explained that this represented the spread to Britain of the Plague of Justinian which had extended in a North Westerly direction from Egypt through Europe, the so-called bubo-plague, which was to reappear in England as the fourteenth century Black Death. Creighton acknowledged that the cause of the disease could only be guessed but that it appeared to him to have originated from some poison in the soil. Further on in the same text, he developed this theory by speculating that localised outbreaks were caused by tainting of the soil and the air by the corruption of corpses insufficiently buried and coffined. At the time when he was writing there was, of course, no knowledge of the roles that rats and their fleas played in the chain of infection.

It is difficult to have any clear idea of when leprosy arrived in England. Some believe that the disease was brought into Britain by the invading Roman armies and support this argument by referring to a fourth century skeleton showing evidence of the condition unearthed from a Romano-British cemetery at Poundbury Camp, Dorchester. Additionally, archeologists have recently excavated what is thought to be England's oldest hospital in Winchester, Hampshire, and analysis of artefacts has provided a date range of AD 960–1030 (i.e. before the Norman conquest of 1066) along with evidence that the establishment was used to treat leprosy (BMJ 2010). However, others believe that leprosy was introduced into England by those returning from the Crusades and it is significant that there is no mention of the condition in the writings of Bede; one feels that he would not have declined the opportunity of commenting on its being brought about by sinning and requiring prayer for a hope of delivery! Certainly it was only after the Norman Conquest that the disease, for about 300 years, seemed to dominate the anxieties of the population as far as health was concerned.

Chapter 2
Infection on the Move

Ask a variety of people what they understand by the term *Renaissance* and you will receive a range of responses but it is likely that they will cluster around the subject matter of what would nowadays be referred to as "high culture", especially that of Italy—painting, sculpture, architecture and music. Classical scholars in England would perhaps emphasise the revival of the study of original Greek and Roman texts rendered available since Caxton set up his printing press at Westminster in 1476. Certainly the printing press transformed European, including English, society. According to McCrum et al. (1986) before 1500 most books were printed in Latin, but between 1500 and 1640 in England alone some 20,000 publications were printed in English, and by 1600 nearly half the population had at least some limited ability to read the texts. With regard to the subject of *this* work, Fraser Brockington (1966) takes the view that, as far as England is concerned, the printing press contributed, *inter alia*, a great deal to the ending of those aspects of the Dark Ages which concerned the lack of understanding of infectious disease in that it allowed the study of the original Classical documents on this topic, rather than having to depend on the monastic trade in manuscripts (which, in his opinion, had been produced in a state of unenlightenment and were full of mistranslations).

However, for the purposes of this study, two other developments were of overwhelming importance: the rediscovery of the essentials of the scientific approach—observation, measurement, recording and interpretation of natural phenomena (including disease), and the extent to which people began to travel—small groups such as seamen venturing beyond Europe for the first time and larger population movements of traders or invading armies.

It is difficult to know where to place bubonic plague within the generally accepted terminology of historical periods in England. Theoretically it came towards the end of the mediaeval period but its arrival in England as the Black Death represented the end point of the westward spread of the disease, originating in Asia and accompanying the major population movements mentioned above. Given that it spanned a period of over 300 years, it could be said to have formed a bridge connecting the late Middle Ages with the Renaissance. It arrived at the Dorset port of Melcombe (now

G. Pollock, *An Epidemiological Odyssey: The Evolution of Communicable Disease Control*, DOI 10.1007/978-94-007-3998-7_2,

part of Weymouth) in August 1348. Its spread through the West Country as far as Bristol, and on to Gloucester and Oxford. was rapid. By the end of that year London had been seriously affected, leading to Parliament being prorogued on the 1st January 1349 and again on 10th March for the reason that "*the pestilence was continuing at Westminster, in the city of London and in other places, more severely than before*" (Rymer 1712).

The disease had arrived in England at a time when the growth of towns with their defensive walls had led to overcrowded and unhygienic urban communities of both people and farm animals, enormously favouring spread of infection. Of course there was as yet no understanding of the cause of the disease. Creighton, even in 1894, felt that, as in the case of the seventh century plague, the Black Death was due to poison in the soil. Not surprisingly, given the ignorance of the times, many believed that the condition represented God's punishment for their sins and looked to prayer as the remedy.

It is difficult to estimate how many died in England at this time. Hatcher (2008) believes that this massively important catastrophe probably wiped out more than four in ten of the population of the known world. However the disease did not inflict a uniform mortality in England; some villages retained their pre-1348 population intact, some were entirely wiped out and there were some where less than a quarter of the inhabitants died (Cartwright 1977). The form in which the disease presented would, of course, have had a major influence on the mortality rate. Pneumonic plague, for example, being both rapidly transmissible and deadly, would have devastated any closed community.

It is perhaps useful to consider how the epidemic affected the town of Coventry, located in the geographical heart of England, as *illustrative* but not necessarily representative of urban populations in the country during the relevant period. Gooder (1998) has drawn attention to some of the features recorded locally. At that time the defensive walls had not yet been built but the town was encircled by a deep protective ditch which approximately followed the same line. Plague probably appeared in Coventry in March 1349 and had spread extensively by April and May. The residents of the town appear to have been more stoical and pragmatic than was generally the case and, in particular, officials stuck to their posts. According to records of property transactions, people did not tend to flee from the city in panic when the Black Death arrived. Nor is there any evidence of self-flagellation or other religious frenzy. The death rate among the local clergy was around 40% and this has been regarded as one guide to the mortality of the town as a whole (although 21% has been another estimate), although it was higher in the poorer and overcrowded areas.

A perhaps unforeseen casualty of the ravages created by the disease was that, as Cartwright (1977) has pointed out, the Church lost a great deal of prestige as the authority to guide on all medical matters. Its claim to offer healing and intercession had not been borne out; the evidence of fearful mortality spoke for itself. Furthermore, according to Hermitage Day (1924), "*The Pope in his palace at Avignon could isolate himself and so find protection against the terrible infection. But the poor in the squalid slums of the towns and the hovels of the countryside were an easy prey to the pestilence.*"

It may be worthwhile pausing for a moment at this point to consider a remark made at a conference on training of epidemiologists held at the Royal Society of Medicine in London in 1970 by Sir James Howie, then Director of the English Public Health Laboratory Service (PHLS),

"*The best way to manage communicable diseases is to discover infections quickly and stop them from spreading.*" One could not have a better or simpler definition of what one would nowadays call integrated surveillance and control. (Perhaps he should have added "*but keep them out of the country in the first place*" which would have been a reasonable definition of quarantine.)

The Black Death probably represented the first spur to concerted action aimed at communicable disease control in Europe. Rosen (1958) has described how some local urban communities found it necessary to establish a few procedures such as:

1. reporting of cases to the Authorities,
2. isolation of cases in their own homes and placing these dwellings under a ban,
3. isolation also of contacts of cases
4. burial of the corpses of cases outside the city walls, with burning of their clothes and fumigation of their houses.

Unfortunately, as Porter (1999) has pointed out, England lagged behind the European Continent in instituting these control measures largely because of its lack of urban political organisations, which meant that there was no authority at local level which could impose the relevant regulations. Not until 1518 were Plague Orders introduced and, as Booker (2008) has described, the country had to wait until 1576 before maritime quarantine was introduced even though, by its not being strictly performed, plague was brought by seamen into the town of Kingston-upon-Hull.

This is not to suggest that there was a lack of expressed *public* concern about the risk. However, in his *Medicine and the Navy 1200–1900*, Keevil (1957) makes it clear that, during the reign of Henry VIII (1509–1547), at no time was any medical opinion sought. Such decisions were left to the King. It was not until 1710 that quarantine against plague was definitely established by an Act of Parliament in Queen Anne's reign. Until that time regulations had had to suffice and, in 1663, such regulations decreed that plague-infested ships approaching London were not to be allowed beyond Gravesend, where they were quarantined for 30 days. This did not, however, prevent the arrival of the Great Plague in the capital 2 years later.

It will be noted that the "package" of public health activities described above by Rosen in relation to mediaeval urban authorities, apart perhaps from some of those listed under 4., still in the twenty-first century may represent a formal requirement in England in certain circumstances concerning infectious diseases although isolation accommodation in hospital would now be generally more relevant. The surveillance element of the above "package" would nowadays be regarded as of the *passive* variety in that the Authorities had to wait until a case was reported before any action could be taken. Not until 1662 was there in England any practice which could be regarded as even a rudimentary form of *active* surveillance and this took a rather unusual and limited form, as is described later.

English history books record that in 1485 the so-called "Wars of the Roses" came to an end when the Duke of Richmond, Henry Tudor, defeated and killed King Richard III at the battle of Bosworth Field, and himself became King Henry VII of England. Shortly after that battle, a severe influenza-like illness broke out amongst the victorious troops. The disease was labelled "the English Sweat" as its principal features, after a sudden and debilitating onset, were high fever and drenching perspiration. The mortality rate was extremely high. One of the puzzling features of this condition was the fact that although it spread rapidly to other parts of England it did not, at that time, invade Scotland, Ireland or the European Continent although subsequent outbreaks of the illness spread widely throughout Northern, Central and Eastern Europe (Rosen 1958). The initial failure to spread could possibly have been due simply to the kind of situation in which those suffering from a disease with a very short incubation period, and which either kills very quickly or at least causes complete prostration, would hardly have been in a position to travel very far.

With regard to the apparent subsequent spread to the Continent, one has to ask: was this really the same disease? There is something bafflingly *non*-specific about a disease which presents as very high fever, perspiration and general bodily aching, with no localising features. In fact, Cartwright and Biddiss (2000) draw attention to the theory that the 1918–1919 pandemic of influenza may have been a recurrence of the English Sweat, not suggesting that the twentieth century pandemic was *not* influenza but that the Sweat may have been the first well-recorded epidemic of influenza originating in, but for some reason localised to, England. Given the ready capacity for influenza viruses to mutate at short notice and exhibit a major change in behaviour, this is not a theory that can be readily dismissed (and has relevance to the situation in which the world has recently found itself regarding the global spread of A/H1N1 "swine flu," initially from Mexico in April 2009).

Hard on the heels of the Black Death and "the Sweat" came a further visitation of quite a different sort to England, also as a result of travel and exploration. In a paper given to the 1986 Spring Conference of the Faculty of Public Health Medicine in London Michael Adler posed an interesting question, suggesting that if students were asked to name a sexually-transmitted disease which had appeared suddenly, was of American origin, caused large numbers of deaths and was regarded by many as a punishment for sins, their response would be "AIDS." In fact the disease being described was syphilis (Adler 1987).

Syphilis was certainly an example of what one would no doubt refer to these days as the "blame culture." The French called it the "Neapolitan disease" whereas Italy referred to the *morbus Gallicus*, a name given to it by the Veronese physician Girolamo Fracastoro in his 1530 poem *Syphilis sive Morbus Gallicus*. The central character in the poem, Syphilis, was a shepherd who was unlucky in his choice of female companion, thereby contracting the disease. Thus Fracastoro gave the world both the name Syphilis and the strong hint that the disease was transmitted sexually. England specifically referred to the French Pox and, as Creighton (1894) has pointed out, when King Henry VIII was in dispute with the Church of Rome, it became socially acceptable to link the disease with alleged scandalous vice among priests, monks and friars. Even Mary Queen of Scots was reported to have forbidden the archbishop to use his spittle in the baptism of her son, James I, as she would not have "a pocky priest" to spit in her child's mouth!

The question of blame was not in any sense restricted to countries. Individuals and lifestyles were picked out in no uncertain manner. As Siena (1998) has described in detail, in sixteenth century England opportunities were readily taken to demonise not only prostitutes but also alehouses, as they encouraged drinking and fornicating among the lower orders, Catholic priests, because of their supposed debauchery with wives and daughters during confession, wet nurses, who were by their very trade presumed to be infectious, and simply *women generally*, whose bodies were conceived as inherently polluting! Throughout the sixteenth century the French pox was said to be the result of God's wrath, although for most of the century it was recognised that sexual intercourse was the most common mode of transmission, the disease being regarded as the Divine punishment for impure sexual contact (Qualtière and Slights 2003).

Making a general point, it is useful to consider two issues concerning the appearance of an apparently new infectious disease: when first someone suggested that the new condition might be infectious, and to what extent this idea was adopted within initially the scientific community and subsequently the general population. The latter issue usually presents far more problems than the former (except, of course, in more recent times of rapid media coverage). Fracastoro's poem was published in 1530 but this was not the first occasion on which the sexual mode of transmission had been proposed. According to McGrew (1985) the Spanish physician Gaspar Torello published in 1497 a tract on the French disease, which he referred to as *pudendagra* and the following year another Spanish physician Francesco Lopez de Villa Lobos in 1498 published a poem concerning "the French pockes" which affected "the parts of shame." It is difficult to know to what extent Fracastoro's literary message was received by the public at large even within his own country, let alone the European population.

The original geographical source of the disease has been much disputed. Fraser Brockington (1966) is only one of many writers who simply accept the circumstantial evidence that the condition was indigenous in the pre-Columbian Native American population and was brought back by the returning Spanish crew in 1493, spreading rapidly within Europe and reaching England in 1497. As Qualtière and Slights (2003) put it, "*The chronological coincidence of the dispersion of Charles VIII of France's multinational of mercenaries and the return of Columbus's crew from the New World convinced many that the new venereal disease was a gift from the Amerindians to Columbus's crew, who carried it back to Europe*." Perhaps understandably, some American writers are reluctant to accept this theory, preferring the alternative explanation that the disease has been in existence throughout human history but that the causative organism underwent some form of mutation towards the end of the fifteenth century. There are, without doubt, many examples of such mutations throughout microbiological history. Also, they can point to a painting by Albrecht Dürer, completed 8 years before Columbus's discovery, which shows a man with lesions suggestive of syphilis.

Some measures were introduced to control its spread once its sexual transmission had been understood. The precedent had actually already been established in

England more than three centuries before the arrival of syphilis itself. In *The Scars of Venus*, Oriel (1994) draws attention to an ordinance of 1162 which prohibited the owners of brothels in Southwark from keeping any woman having the sickness of *brenning* (burning), presumably gonorrhoea or some other form of urethritis associated with painful urination.

Siena (1998) has set out some of the measures which were adopted in sixteenth century England. The ready recognition of prostitutes as a main source of infection justified the closure of public brothels by order of King Henry VIII in 1546 and an anonymous practitioner even suggested in a pamphlet *Profulacticon: Or Some Considerations of a Notable Expedient To root out the French Pox From the English Nation* that those affected be transported to the West Indies! Both anti-alehouse and anti-wet nurse movements were launched by Calvinists, against a background of the promotion of monogamous marriage in contrast to the dangers of consorting with prostitutes. Perhaps the most extreme reaction was an attempt to isolate sufferers, rather as had happened to lepers in mediaeval times (Porter 1999). The rich were to remain in home isolation whereas the poor were driven out of the community. A law of James IV of Scotland ruled that sufferers had to depart from Edinburgh to reside on the nearby island of Inchkeith (Oriel 1994).

Fracastoro (1546) did much more than throw light on the spread of simply one sexually transmitted disease. Sixteen years after his elegant allegorical poem concerning the luckless shepherd he published *De Contagione et Contagiosis Morbis et Eorum Curatione* written in three books: the first of the notion of contagion, the second applying this idea to a variety of infectious diseases, and the third suggesting possible treatments for these diseases. He was, of course, not the first to postulate the idea of contagion. As mentioned earlier, leprosy had been recognised in Old Testament times as a condition which could spread if the diseased were not isolated from the general community and Sushruta in 600 BC India had produced clinical evidence for the ability of the disease to be carried from a sufferer to a healthy person (Buhier 1886). What Fracastoro did was to suggest in detail how these communicable diseases were actually transmitted from person to person by "seeds of contagion" in three different kinds of situation: "*The first infects by direct contact only, the second does the same but in addition leaves fomes, thirdly there is a kind of contagion that infects at a distance.*" Even here, he was not the first to come up with the idea of minute animate creatures which could spread through the air and enter the body through the nose or mouth as Marcus Terentius Varro had done just that in 36 BC.

Fracastoro's work was widely discussed by his contemporaries but, although it clearly provided the basis for research which would lead eventually to modern epidemiological methods, not all his colleagues accepted his conclusions (Nutton 1990). Nevertheless, although his ideas spread first only within Northern Italy, by the middle of the sixteenth century it was clear that they had influenced public health policies in Paris and London.

Trading contacts with countries in Asia and the Eastern Mediterranean along with a variety of military conflicts continued to result in the importation of new infections to Europe, although new diseases were not necessarily recognised quickly or were sometimes themselves apparently confused with other, existing, febrile conditions. However McGrew (1985) accepts the evidence that epidemic typhus fever was brought to Europe in the late fifteenth century during the siege of Granada, the infection carried by troops arriving from Cyprus.

However the symptoms of this disease were not very specific—essentially high fever and prostration, with or without rash—and confusion with other conditions exhibiting high temperatures persisted. For example, when the first international conference took place in Paris in 1851 to discuss the question of quarantine many delegates are reported to have been able to distinguish between typhus fever and plague. And in England, as Rosen (1958) points out, it was not until the late nineteenth century that typhus fever was officially separated from other "fevers" for record purposes. Furthermore the fact that the disease was transmitted by body lice was not recognised until 1911 meant that, until that time, other than appreciating the risks of persons having to live in closely confined, none too clean, conditions (such as soldiers, seamen and prisoners) there was no understanding of the precise mode of transmission. It could be considered a bitter irony arising from this ignorance that, in the so-called "Black Assizes" in Cambridge in 1522, prisoners from the filthy gaol who were brought to court passed the infection to the judge on the bench, with a fatal outcome for the latter. Spread of typhus fever could not, of course, be totally prevented in wartime. Up to and including the Second World War, and even at the end of the latter conflict, older readers may recall seeing newsreel footage in the cinemas of persons in camps for European displaced persons being "deloused" by having insecticide powder insufflated throughout their clothing.

Yet another serious infection brought to England by travellers in the early sixteenth century was smallpox, originating possibly in China or India. According to Creighton (1894) the earliest references occur in letters written in 1514 and 1518. For example in a letter of March 3rd 1514 Peter Martyr indicated that King Henry VIII had suffered from a fever which was referred to as "la petitte verolle" (the *small* pox, to distinguish it from "la grosse verolle," the Great or French Pox). Some believe that the disease existed from earliest times and McGrew (1985) suggests that the earliest identifiable case was the Egyptian pharaoh Ramses V who died about 1160 BC, although neither Greek or Hebrew sources record cases with a similar picture of fever and the characteristic rash. Furthermore Cartwright and Biddiss (2000) point out that no depiction of a pock-mark has been found on any representation of the human features from those periods although they accept that such disfigurement could have been deliberately omitted for aesthetic reasons, perhaps an early example of "airbrushing!"

Most medical historians accept that smallpox was identified as a clearly recognisable clinical entity only when the Persian physician referred to as Rhazes, or Al Rhazi, distinguished it from measles around AD 900. To some, it may seem strange that smallpox, remembered until its eradication in the late 1970s as a "killer" disease much to be feared, could be confused with what they may still regard as a trifling childhood condition. Such perplexity is based on three false assumptions. Firstly, smallpox in sixteenth century England was not always the lethal disease that it was to become in later centuries and could almost have been regarded as a routine affliction of childhood; Cartwright (1977) makes the point that "smallpox and measles" was a common diagnosis at that time applied to a single illness. Secondly, measles could, and did, cause devastation when introduced into new susceptible communities or populations with no pre-existing immunity, perhaps the best illustration of this phenomenon being when the disease reached the Faroe Islands in 1846 affecting over three-quarters of the population, and a case fatality of 1.7%. Lastly, even today in unvaccinated communities in England, according to Salisbury et al. (2006) measles can have serious complications—otitis media (7–9%), pneumonia (1–6%) and convulsions (1 in 200).

The prevention, control and eventual eradication of smallpox were almost completely dependent on the introduction of vaccination. However this procedure and the manner in which its introduction was handled professionally and politically in the nineteenth century are considered to have had a profound influence on the British attitude to vaccination and immunisation procedures generally, resulting in all such arrangements being totally voluntary and informal, unlike e.g. the United States, France, Malta or Poland. Because of this, details of the fight against smallpox and the eventual victory are dealt with in Chap. 8.

Bubonic plague had not disappeared from England after the main visitation of the Black Death in the fourteenth century. In fact, according to Creighton (1894), for the 1,000-year period from 664, when the country was caught up in the Northward sweep of the Plague of Justinian, through the Black Death itself, until 1666, when the disease was extinguished at the end of the Great Plague of London, the condition had been smouldering on, flaring up in isolated and limited outbreaks. The overall impact of the disease on English social life was colossal. As Porter (1999) has described, the Black Death killed about one third of the population of England and led to the break-up of the feudal system by creating a shortage of agricultural workers, who were thereby able to move around the country in search of better-paid employment.

The disease demanded that society take action to protect the community by some form of organised response and, as stated earlier, England eventually followed the example of the European continent in terms of civic protection and quarantine. An extract from the Coventry Council Book for 1665 (Fig. 2.1) gives details of an Order to prevent the bringing of the plague to that city (City Record Office). Predictably, throughout the country, physicians and "quacks" were much in evidence, peddling secret remedies. One such, "Goddard's Drop," was sold to King Charles II for £6,000, even though this proved to be simply mixtures such as spirit of raw silk rectified with oil of cinnamon. Dr Goddard was a member of the council of the Royal Society but his own personal remedy for the catastrophe was to flee the area (Creighton 1894)! This latter course of action was practised by many who were rich enough to afford to do so, hence the profusion of "Little Londons," such as the one at Tadley, Hampshire, localities up to about 50 miles from London which were settled by those escaping the Great Plague of 1665.

In Scotland, too, the wealthy took appropriate evasive action, although this was not always successful. In the well-known traditional song "Betsy Bell and Mary Gray" the story is told of two daughters of country gentlemen in the neighbourhood

PLAGUE

An Order to prevent the bringing of the plague of pestilence into this Citie

For as much as it hathe pleased the Lord (for the Sinnes of this Nation) to afflict the same in the chief Cities thereof and other places, with that heavie disease of plague and pestilence, which this last week hath much increased.

And wee, the Maior and Aldermen of this Citie (to whome the safeguard of this Citie is committed by the kings Maj) being desirous to use our best care and diligence to prevent the bringing of the plague of pestilence and other contagious diseases into this Citie and these parts, as neere as we can, have therefore considered and set downe these ensuing orders following.

That the respective Constables of this Citie during the time of this infection, do in their respective wards from henceforth warne so many inhabitants of this Citie in their severall Wards to watch and ward everie night and day in theire own persons or to send sufficient able men in their rooms: And in default of such watch and ward the respective Constables to call them out to watch and warde in theire owne persons.

And that everie night one Constable do in his owne person watch everie night, which they are to take by turns and one Constable to Ward everie day.

The watch to begin at eight o'clock at night and the Ward to relieve them on the next morning at six of the clock and continue till eight o'clock at night.

In anie inhabitant of this Citie receive any person o0r goods from London or other infected places, then a Warden to be set at their doore to keepe them in and in case they be able, to paie the Warden, which, if they refuse, to deny them. If poore, let them have to sustaine life but let them smart.

In any constable or other person disobey this order, to be committed to prison, which necessitie requires.

Given at the said Citie under our hand and the Common Seale of the said Citie in such way ordained, the 22nd July Anno Domini 1665.

Fig. 2.1 Extract from the Council Book for 1665: Reference, A14B; City Record Office

of Perth who, to escape the infection, built themselves a bower by a stream and had food delivered to them by a young man who was very romantically attached to both of them. Unfortunately this young man also unintentionally delivered the infection to them and they both died:

O Betsy Bell and Mary Gray
They were twa bonnie lasses
They biggit a bower on yon burn-brae
And theekit it o'er wi' rashes
They theekit it o'er wi rashes green
They theekit it o'er wi' heather
But the pest cam' frae the borough's toun
And slew them baith thegither
They thocht to lie in Methven kirkyard
Amang their noble kin
But they maun lie in Dronach-Haugh
And beik forenenst the sun.

Perhaps an even more bitter irony was in evidence by what happened in the Derbyshire village of Eyam in 1665 when the plague reached their locality via some old clothes sent from London. Instead of fleeing the scene, the villagers were persuaded by the vicar to lock themselves in the church. Almost all died in this heroic demonstration of the possibility of breaking the chain of infection (Fraser Brockington 1966).

Chapter 3
The Impact of Cholera

From 1949, on the facade of No. 18 Sackville Street, London, until 1965 (when the house was demolished to make way for commercial developments), there was a commemorative plaque which read:

> **JOHN SNOW 1813–1858, physician and specialist anaesthetist who discovered that cholera is water-borne, lived here** (Galbraith 2002).

Dr Snow, who was in fact the first specialist anaesthetist in the country, is usually also regarded as the country's first epidemiologist (although he was not the first to adopt an epidemiological approach, as is shown below) and it is in this latter role that he is of critical importance to this piece of work. But before his unique contribution to understanding "*the Mode of Communication of Cholera*" (as he named his 1849 pamphlet) can be described in any meaningful sense, one has to have some idea of the means by which information concerning cases of illness or causes of deaths was collected and analysed, and for that one has to go back a further two centuries.

Many professional people, famous or otherwise, have had unusual hobbies. Prime Minister Winston Churchill enjoyed building brick walls; Ken Livingstone, the former Mayor of London, kept a collection of newts as pets; a colonel whom I knew personally during my army National Service was skilled at making fine fishing rods. John Graunt, a prosperous seventeenth century haberdasher with a mathematical turn of mind found fascination in examining the figures showing the numbers of deaths, and their reported causes, in London. He compiled and published his comments on these as *The Natural and Political Observations upon the Bills of Mortality* in 1662, drawing upon the figures for the previous 30 years.

In the Preface to his publication Graunt explained why he had embarked on this study:

> *Having been born and bred in the City of London, and having always observed that most of them who took in the weekly Bills of Mortality made little other use of them than to look at the foot, how the Burials increase or decrease. Now I thought that the Wisdom of our City had certainly designed the laudable practice of takeing and distributing these Accompts, for other and greater uses than those above-mentioned, or at least some other uses might*

G. Pollock, *An Epidemiological Odyssey: The Evolution of Communicable Disease Control*, DOI 10.1007/978-94-007-3998-7_3,

be made of them.......................comparing Year, Season, Parish or other Division of the City and of all the Diseases and Casualties happening in each of them respectively (Graunt 1662).

Without realising it, he was carrying out the first study which could be described as genuinely epidemiological, i.e. the examination of patterns of disease in a community in relation to person, time and place. Additionally, he was carefully observing certain demographic issues, such as the excess of male over female births and the fact that urban mortality figures were greater than their rural counterparts.

The field-workers who collected the raw data at Parish level were known as "searchers:"

"*When any one dies, either by tolling or ringing of a bell or by bespeaking of a grave, the same is known to the searchers who hereupon repair to the place where the dead Corps lies, and by view of the same, and by other enquiries, they examine by what*
Disease, or Casualty, the Corps died.

However, Graunt appeared to have rather a poor opinion of *female* searchers who:

"*after the Mist of a Cup of Ale, and the Bribe of a Two-groat fee, instead of the one given them*"were likely to be unable to record the cause of death with any degree of accuracy, or to be party to concealing the fact that death had been due to syphilis! An exception, in his view, to such situations could occur:

"*In many of these cases the Searchers are able to report the Opinion of the Physician who was with the Patient.*"

He understood, but did not have much sympathy with, the reluctance to name syphilis as a cause of death:

We finde one Casualty in our Bills, of which although there be daily talk, there is little effect. much like our abhorrence of Toads and Snakes..........and this Casualty is the French-Pox, gotten, for the most part, not so much by the intemperate use of Venery (which rather causes the Gowt) as of many common Women............We shall therefore shew, that the Pox is not as the Toads and Snakes afore-mentioned, but of a quite contrary nature, together with the reason, why it appears otherwise.

Reference was made in Chap. 2 to the development of *passive* surveillance during the period of the Black Death, i.e. cases being reported to the Authorities so that the latter could respond by isolating such cases and their contacts and, among other things, placing their dwellings under a ban and fumigating them. The weakness of these arrangements lay in the fact that the Authorities could take appropriate action only when someone had reported a case in the first instance. The main significance of Graunt's diligent enquiries and published findings was that he had demonstrated a rudimentary form of *active* surveillance of a defined population in that he had taken the initiative by searching for information rather than waiting for someone to report it to him. The fact that the recorded data concerned only deaths did, of course, represent a significant limitation of its value, but he had nevertheless been able to comment on patterns of disease in a particular community, relating these to place, time and other circumstance—in other words the essence of the epidemiological approach, which still applies in the twenty-first century. Furthermore, as Rosen (1958) has pointed out, Graunt had shown, by testing the reliability of his findings, that even imperfect data, if interpreted with care and thoughtfulness, could yield valuable information—once more a central tenet of modern epidemiology.[1]

However nearly 200 years was to pass before Dr John Snow skillfully demonstrated the practical application of the epidemiological method in elucidating the means of spread of cholera in London, as is described below.

It is believed that cholera had been endemic in the Indian Sub-continent for at least 2,000 years but it was not until the era of travel associated with the Renaissance that there were reports of an epidemic disease whose symptoms were those of cholera, and no cases appeared in Europe until the nineteenth century (McGrew 1985).

In 1829 there was much concern in England over the relentless Westward spread of the disease through Russia and Poland. However this was not the first occasion on which the Government had expressed great anxiety over the possible spread of an epidemic from the Continent to England. In 1720, alarmed at the opportunities which plague might have to be carried by ship to British ports from Marseille, which was experiencing a severe epidemic, George I's government commissioned Dr Richard Mead to prepare a report as a matter of urgency, offering advice and guidance. The classic document which resulted, *A Short Discourse concerning Pestilential Contagion and the Methods used to prevent it*, covered all aspects of public health control including case-finding, isolation and maritime quarantine, in effect emphasising recommendations which, as described in Chap. 2, had been around in England since the sixteenth century (and even earlier, in mediaeval times, on the Continent of Europe). Mead's intention was, if at all possible, to keep plague from gaining access to the country in the first place:

> *As it is a satisfaction to know that the plague is not a native of our country..........we must find out means to keep ourselves clear from it..........by obliging ships that come from infected places to perform quarantine. Near to our several ports, there should be lazarettos built in convenient places for the reception of both men and goods. The sick, if there be any, should be kept in houses remote from the sound* (Mead 1720).

It is interesting to note that Richard Mead appeared to share John Graunt's somewhat sexist views regarding searchers:

> *Instead of ignorant old women, who are generally appointed searchers in Parishes to enquire what diseases people die of, that Office should be committed to understanding and diligent men, whose business it should be, as soon as they find any have died after an uncommon manner, particularly with livid spots, buboes or carbuncles, to give notice thereof to the Council of Health who should immediately send skilful physicians to examine the suspected bodies...........*

In fact plague did not spread from France to England on that occasion and it seems reasonable to assume that the implementation of Mead's advice on maritime quarantine may have played a part in this.

[1] Italian historians are keen to point out that Bills of Mortality were created in Italy about 200 years before this happened in London (Milan in 1452 and Mantua in 1496) but the reason for their being less well known is that there was never any Italian equivalent of John Graunt to study them! (Cipolla 1976).

Understandably, then, Mead's recommendations became highly relevant once more against the background of the growing anxiety over the possibility of cholera reaching England from Europe, referred to above. Here was another opportunity to isolate England from the Continent and thereby protect its population. Accordingly in April 1831 the Admiralty issued orders for a strict quarantine of all arrivals from Russia at British ports (Creighton 1894) and a Central Board of Health was set up by Royal Proclamation on 21 June under the aegis of the Privy Council. At its first meeting the members wished to know what, if any, modifications should be made to the Rules and Regulations of Quarantine of 1825, what general rules should govern the separation of the sick from the healthy, and what measures were required to prevent spread of the disease should it gain access to this country (Fraser Brockington 1965).

It was, in fact, just as well that the last-mentioned issue was raised as, at the end of July and in August of that year, the port of Sunderland and the adjoining villages and farms in the Wear Valley were affected by the disease which, at first, was thought to be simply an indigenous form of diarrhoea although many of the cases seemed "unusually malignant" (Creighton 1894). "*One case, a girl of twelve named Hazard, who resided on the Fish Quay and who was well enough on Sunday 16th of October to have been twice at church, nevertheless was seized in the middle of the night with appalling symptoms and died on the Monday afternoon. A few doors off, on the same quay, lived a keelman named Sproat, aged sixty, who was seized with rigor, cramps, vomiting and purging; after a few days of such symptoms he died on the 26th of October*" (Dixon 1832).

Creighton believed that the means by which cholera entered Sunderland had never been traced but he was aware that deaths from cholera had occurred among the crews of Sunderland ships lying at Cronstadt and Riga. Furthermore it was his opinion that the quarantine station in the Wear was far from effective as it was higher up the river than the loading moorings so that suspected ships had to pass through a crowd of ordinary shipping to get to it. Having entered the country through this North-East port the disease spread widely, causing about 22,000 deaths within 9 months (Macnamara 1892).

The significance of the country's "armour" being penetrated in this way was profound. Quarantine could no longer be depended upon as a guarantee of the nation's immunity and the issues raised by the Central Board of Health, if such a contingency were to befall the country, became of immediate relevance. Even without the Central Board's encouragement, cities, towns and other communities clearly recognised the urgent need to protect their own populations and, as a result, local boards of health were rapidly coming into being, formally constituted by Orders in Council. These local boards were to consist of members of the medical profession, clergymen and leading citizens who would maintain contact with the Central Board, which would be prepared to offer some guidance on dealing with patients and their belongings (Cartwright and Biddiss 2000).

Not surprisingly, the Privy Council received requests for such authority initially from ports such as Barmouth, Bristol, Hull, Manchester, Newcastle-upon-Tyne, North Shields, Rochester and Sunderland itself (Fraser Brockington 1965). The Illustration, listing the Recommendations of the first meeting of the Sunderland

Sunderland BOARD OF HEALTH,

Constituted by an Order of Council.

At a Meeting of the Board, on the 28th Day of Nov. 1831,

IT was Resolved, 1st, That it is the duty of every Medical Practitioner, when called to a Pauper Patient labouring under Cholera, to use his best endeavours to persuade his Patient to consent to be removed to the Cholera Hospital without delay; and in the event of such Patient refusing to comply with that advice, it shall then be the duty of the Medical Attendant to give immediate notice to the nearest of the undermentioned Medical Inspectors, who have been appointed by the Board, viz.—Dr. Miller, Dr. Hazlewood, Dr. Ogden, and Mr. Torbock, and who shall, with all convenient speed, visit the said Patient; and should he see fit, he shall urge the instant removal of the Patient, and if that cannot be done, to report on such case to the Board.

2nd, That the Medical Inspectors be empowered to call on any Medical Practitioner for a daily state of his Cholera Patients, not coming under the denomination of Paupers, should either such Patients or their Medical Attendant refuse to allow the Medical Inspectors, to see them.

3rd, That all Medical Practitioners and Inspectors be required to comply strictly with the foregoing Resolutions and Directions; and that in case of any omission or neglect in carrying the same into full effect, immediate information thereof be given to this Board, in order that a report thereon may be transmitted to Government.

4th, That the Board do state, in proof of the superior advantage of early Hospital Treatment, that out of a Family of five Persons attacked with Cholera, the only Individuals who recovered were the two conveyed to, and attended at, the Hospital.

MEMORANDUM.—That the Privy Council have ordered that, in future, no examination, after death, of persons conveyed to the Hospital, shall take place.

5th, That the Secretary be requested to transmit a Copy of the foregoing Resolutions and Order to each Medical Gentleman, and that Copies be generally circulated in these Towns.

By Order of the Board,

GEO. STEPHENSON,

SECRETARY.

Board of Health conveys a clear picture of the determination of the officials of that town to do all in their power to protect their local community. In all, between 1831 and 1834, around 800 local health boards were set up in England. Some local authorities, mainly those far inland, did not move with such urgency. For example Coventry (as far from any coast as could be imagined) did not have a local health board until 1849, i.e. not until the year of the *second* major cholera epidemic (Midland Daily Telegraph 7th September 1937), even though the local public health report for the City in the 1831 Census described its atmosphere as "tainted and impure in the extreme, with the working classes involved in watchmaking or silk and ribbon weaving having to work in confined, ill-ventilated rooms" although its suburban districts seemed "mild and very healthy" .

At first sight it might seem that English municipalities had at last caught up with their Continental counterparts, whose arrangements had existed since mediaeval times. It is certainly true that both had been motivated by the enlightened self-interest of local security and both were also governed by rules to attempt to achieve this. However there was an important difference: municipal health boards and councils of health in Europe came into existence independently when the individual local authority deemed this necessary, whereas the first "crop" of English health boards was created almost simultaneously in relation to one specific threat to health and, linked to the Centre for both formal authority and professional guidance, **they constituted the early stages of a network which was to become the country's first nation-wide system of public health**.

There were, no doubt, many other reasons for England appearing to have lagged behind the European Continent in setting up municipal organisations for the prevention and control of disease locally. Fraser Brockington (1966), for example, took the view that, whereas the political organisation of the Continent was already reformed, England's had yet to be carried out. Furthermore he felt that, between 1800 and 1830, England had preoccupations with political issues rather than with questions of health and that it took the cholera threat to alter the priorities. Certainly readers of George Eliot's 1872 novel *Middlemarch*, set in the English Midlands during the period leading up to the Reform Act of 1832, will recall the intensity and heat of the political debates, and the difficulties which the young, idealistic doctor experienced in having his plea for a local fever hospital heard. (I was reminded of this when I came to work in Coventry, considered by many to be at or near the location of "Middlemarch", in 1963 as my duties included working with Dr Joseph Galpine, the infectious diseases consultant, in Whitley Isolation Hospital in the city—almost certainly the kind of institution which Eliot's hero would have had in mind for the locality, and no doubt brought into being as a result of strong advocacy on the part of such an individual in real life.)

It has to be realised, of course, that at this point these control measures were purely empirical as, not only was there no general understanding of the mechanism by which cholera spread, there were still many who were resistant to the idea that diseases were, in fact, communicable. Although the notion of contagion had its supporters, there were also those who favoured the idea that particular weather conditions (epidemic constitution) and/or unpleasant smells (miasma) could cause disease.

Although the latter views may now seem absurd, some of these ideas had existed since the time of Hippocrates, and one could readily accept that a foul stench arising from poor sanitation could be interpreted as a cause of ill-health. Also, the anti-contagionists could truthfully point out, quarantine measures had not prevented the spread of disease either in England or within the European Continent (Porter 1999).

Eighteen months after the epidemic came to an end in December 1832, the Central Board of Health was discontinued but many local boards of health remained in existence as people had seen the value of a local body which could not only deal with cases of cholera but could represent a local democratic body with a responsibility for a general oversight of health matters in its area.

However the year 1832 was also one of critical importance for the development of public health in England for a quite separate reason; as in a relay race, one process was beginning to pick up speed just as another appeared to be running out of steam! At the same time as the evidence suggested that the threat of cholera had subsided, so that expensive administrative organisations such as the Central Board of Health could be dispensed with, the Government was in the process of setting up a Royal Commission to enquire into the working of the by then outdated Poor Law so that recommendations could be made for ameliorating the lot of labouring people. The Government had been prompted to respond to major social unrest, its concern having been intensified by the riots occurring in the worst slum areas of industrial towns during the run-up to the 1832 Reform Act (Cartwright and Biddiss 2000).

A lawyer, Edwin Chadwick, was recruited to assist with this work and in the process of investigating the problems he came to the conclusion that poverty in working class families was largely brought about by disease leading to incapacity or death affecting the male breadwinner, thereby leaving a dependent family. Therefore, he concluded, the costs of public relief could actually be cut by preventing disease (Lewis 1991). By observing the association between the incidence of fevers and the combination of massive overcrowding, inadequate waste disposal and polluted water he accepted the miasma theory without question. As Porter (1997) has pointed out, it was perhaps easy to believe in the miasma theory as the overwhelming impact of these overcrowded towns at that time was their stench which must have seemed strong and foul enough to kill or at least produce vomiting. Accordingly, Chadwick's famous 1842 Report "*on the sanitary condition of the labouring population*" argued that the country would gain enormously by taking steps to create a more hygienic environment and that the most useful way forward was to apply the technical skills necessary to develop major civil engineering projects leading to proper drainage and sewerage, improved water supplies and effective house and street cleansing (McGrew 1985).

However Chadwick, although he had no great opinion of physicians in private practice, also accepted the need for a *salaried* medical input in specifying the nature, location and likely course of the disease:

> *That for the promotion of the means necessary to prevent disease, it would be good economy to appoint a district medical officer, independant* (sic) *of private practice, and with securities of special qualifications, and (with) responsibilities to initiate sanitary measures and reclaim the execution of the law* (Chadwick 1842).

In the above quotation it can clearly be seen that Chadwick was bringing focus to bear on five critical issues: 1. *that public health should be seen as a local matter (i.e. at "district" level);* 2. *that a "public" doctor (i.e. one relating to a community rather than to separate individuals) should play a key role;* 3. *that this medical practitioner should possess special qualifications relating to the field of work;* 4. *that he should have formal accountability to his local community; and* 5. *that the execution of his duties should have the backing of the law.* **Thus, as stated by Chave** (1984)**, the idea of the Medical Officer of Health was first conceived**.

The first English Public Health Act was passed in 1848, replacing the Poor Law Commission with a new General Board of Health, and permitting but not requiring local authorities to appoint a Surveyor, an Inspector of Nuisances and a Medical Officer of Health, and giving powers to undertake work including sewerage and water supply systems. Interestingly, the appointment or removal of the Medical Officer of Health was subject to the approval of the General Board of Health (Frazer 1950). As far as his removal was concerned, the fact that this could achieved only with the consent of the Board represented the beginning of what was soon to be referred to as "security of tenure." (The essentially permissive nature of this Act was emphasised; it was not until 1872 that legislation was enacted *requiring* local authorities to appoint such staff and to undertake appropriate work.)

The City of Liverpool had not waited for national legislation, having acted independently in 1847 under a local Act, appointing a local general practitioner, William Duncan, as Officer of Health, the first in the country. By virtue of his appointment, Dr Duncan was required to inspect and report from time to time on the health aspects of the Borough's environment and more specifically, as outlined in the relevant Clause:

> *to ascertain the existence of diseases, more especially epidemics increasing the rate of mortality, and to point out the existence of any nuisances or other local causes which are likely to originate and maintain such diseases, and injuriously affect inhabitants of the said Borough, and to take cognisance of the fact of the existence of any contagious disease and so to point out the most efficacious means for checking and preventing the spread of such diseases* (John 1987).

The City of London took similar action in the following year, also using a local Act in advance of the national legislation, appointing John Simon, a surgeon from St Thomas's Hospital as Medical Officer of Health, and during the next 25 years most of the major towns made similar appointments. Simon's formal responsibilities were similar to those outlined above for Dr Duncan but his professional inclination was to look beyond the physical environment to examine the question of disease itself. It quickly became clear to him that he needed as early, as accurate and as full information as was possible about every fluctuation in the health of the City and to do this he proposed to use outside bodies. (Lambert 1963).

In this connection, applications of important vital statistics were becoming available through the efforts of William Farr, appointed Compiler of Statistical Abstracts in 1838. Farr's originality was demonstrated by collecting relevant facts, assembling and evaluating them, and reporting them to responsible health authorities as well as to the general public. Many of his reports were used to support campaigns against disease, beginning with his intensive study of the cholera returns during the 1848–1849 epidemic (Farr/Humphreys 1885).

The statutory duties of the Medical Officer of Health, as spelt out initially for William Duncan and John Simon, represented a situation in which the Government could be seen to be feeling its way towards minimising the impact of potential hazards of the local environment. They clearly had a particular focus on the control of infectious diseases and, in the circumstances, it would have been difficult to conceive of any other approach. Later national legislation had the intention of clarifying and widening these responsibilities, for example in an Order of 1910 for local authorities outside London the wording was:

> *[The Medical Officer of Health] shall inform himself, as far as practicable, respecting all influences affecting or threatening to affect injuriously the public health within the District. He shall inquire into and ascertain by such means are at his disposal the causes, origin and distribution of diseases within the District, and ascertain to what extent the same have depended on conditions capable of removal or mitigation.*

This gave individual Medical Officers of Health considerable scope, and the general approach adopted by most (including myself when Medical Officer of Health of the City of Coventry) could be summed up as "find out whatever may be adversely affecting the health of the population of your district and deal with it as best you can." This clearly meant achieving results by influence, as much as by authority, and depended on securing the goodwill and practical support of a large number of persons, only beginning with doctors, nurses and the personnel currently known as environmental health officers, and going on to include teachers, social workers, the media and local politicians. Fortunately, the way forward had been well demonstrated by John Simon.

The 1848 Public Health Act had encouraged the creation of local boards of health, but now certain criteria had to be satisfied including the expressed wishes of the local population in the form of a petition. By the year 1849, for example, "*the Coventry Local Board of Health had become the responsible body for the health of the citizens, having successfully petitioned the General Board of Health for such authority, and no greater task could have been set in the early days of its establishment for the City once again found itself in the deadly grip of the cholera scourge in which 269 citizens died. The scourge became rampant and relief agencies were organised in all parts of the town. The cholera first showed itself about the end of July in the Harnall Lane area where the houses were for the most part small and crowded, while the number of inmates was far greater than was consistent with hygiene. Further, in close proximity was a stagnant ditch like a miniature moat, while in the surface drainage heaps of refuse accumulated to such an extent as to impede progress along the thoroughfare*" (Midland Daily Telegraph 7th September 1937). There was even a special form of prayer introduced on Sunday 16th September 1849, to be used in all churches and chapels, "during the prevalence of cholera in this country, for obtaining pardon of our sins" (Tomlinson 1849).

The year 1849 was also significant, in a national sense, in that it produced John Snow's first publication on the epidemiology of cholera, his famous *On the Mode of Communication of Cholera*, in the form of (to use his own modest phrase) a "slender pamphlet." His introduction to the subject had occurred relatively early in adult life as when he was 14 years of age he was apprenticed to William Hardcastle, a surgeon in Newcastle-upon-Tyne, just as cholera was reaching that area following its importation through the port of Sunderland in 1831. The local epidemic which followed involved 1,330 cases and caused 801 deaths (Galbraith 2002). At a local coal-mine in Killingworth, miners were experiencing a particularly high death rate and Hardcastle sent his apprentice to do what he could for the miners and their families, although the young man had to accept eventually that he could make no impact on this localized epidemic. Nevertheless this made him all the more determined to try to gain a greater understand of the disease (Adler 2004).

By 1838 John Snow had become a qualified medical practitioner and was living at 54 Frith Street, Soho, London. After years of building up a private practice (mainly as an anaesthetist) he acquired additional medical qualifications from the University of London and took an active part in medical societies dealing with the scientific side of medicine (Galbraith 2002). It was natural, therefore, that he should pursue his interest in cholera when the disease recurred in London in 1848.

In his "slender pamphlet" he made it clear straightaway that, in his view, the question of the communicability of the disease was not at issue:

> *It is propagated by human intercourse. Its progress along the great channels of that intercourse and the very numerous instances both in this country and abroad in which cholera dates its commencement in a town or village previously free from it to the arrival and illness of a person coming from a place in which the disease was prevalent seem to leave no room for doubting its communicability* (Snow 1849).

He accepted, however, that this view was disputed by some but he dismissed such arguments on the general philosophical principle that belief based on lack of evidence should not override evidence of a positive kind. He also refuted any ideas which allowed the theory of communicability but rested on the belief that emanations from the sick persons caused contagion by e.g. being inhaled and absorbed by the blood in the lungs, as might be the case in other illnesses. He observed that symptoms in cholera related initially to the alimentary canal and that subsequent clinical features could be traced to that original affection. He was quick to spot the likely source of infection from the patient:

> *Having rejected effluvia to the poisoning of the blood in the first instance, and being led to the conclusion that the disease is communicated by something that acts directly on the alimentary canal, the excretions of the sick at once suggest themselves as containing some material which, being accidentally swallowed, might attach itself to the mucous membrane of the small intestine and there multiply itself by the appropriateness of surrounding matter in value of molecular changes going on within it.*

He went on to offer the analogy of worm infestation by ingestion of ova, and expressed concern over the difficulties of avoiding being infected by a patient:

> *That a portion of the ejection or dejection must often be swallowed by healthy persons is, however, a matter of necessity. The latter are voided with such suddenness and force that clothes and bedding scarcely fail to become soiled. Hence these become attached to the hands of the person nursing the patient and are unconsciously swallowed unless care be taken to wash the hands before partaking of food.*

Having discussed how secondary cases might arise from the original patient he now moved on to consider how the infection came into a community in the first place. His first observation concerned the likely role of water:

> *Cholera may be widely disseminated by the emptying of sewers into the drinking water of the community and as far as the writer's inquiries have extended, he has found that in most towns in which the malady has prevailed to an unusual extent this means of communication has existed.*

He gave examples of the above situation occurring in Glasgow, Dumfries and Maxwelltown in Scotland, and also commented on the fact that in the cholera epidemic of 1832 the disease had been much more prevalent in the South and East Districts of London, supplied by water from the much contaminated rivers Thames and Lea, than other parts of the metropolis which had different water sources. He then went on to describe the outcome of some of his more detailed studies in different parts of London, drawing attention to the remarkable association between the local occurrence of cholera cases with situations in which water was being contaminated by the contents of drains and cesspools. However he concentrated on what he felt was the large-scale issue, namely the risks from major sources of pollution in the rivers which provided London's drinking water, showing that once again cholera was more prevalent in the South and East Districts, supplied by the Thames and Lea, than in the North and Central Districts, whose water was derived from Hertfordshire, and the West Districts, who enjoyed the privilege of water from the Thames several miles upstream from London.

He presented these findings with due modesty but with an underlying sense of conviction:

> *These opinions respecting the cause of cholera are brought forward, not as matters of certainty, but as containing a greater amount of probability in their favour than any other, in the present state of our knowledge.*

His conviction led him to assert that cholera might be checked and kept at bay by simple measures such as careful washing of the hands and avoiding drinking water from sources into which drains and sewers emptied themselves or, if necessary, filtering and boiling the water before use.

Snow did not expect his findings, at this stage, to be universally accepted and indeed this proved to be the case. William Farr fully supported Snow's recommendations but did not yet rule out miasma as a contributory cause of the disease (Pelling 1978).

Snow's next opportunity to shed light on the source and spread of cholera occurred in 1854 when his own district of Soho was affected by a sudden and violent local outbreak beginning on the 31st August. As he himself described it (Snow 1855): "*The most terrible outbreak of cholera which ever occurred in this kingdom is probably that which took place in Broad Street, Golden Square and the adjoining streets. Within two hundred and fifty yards of the spot where Cambridge Street joins Broad Street, there were upwards of five hundred fatal attacks of cholera in ten days.*"

Because of his particular interest, he began to engage in what is usually referred to these days as "shoe-leather epidemiology," first ascertaining at which local addresses deaths had occurred, then enquiring from relations of the victims the source of their water supply. He soon came to the conclusion that the pump at the heart of the epidemic was situated at the corner of Broad Street and Cambridge Street. Accordingly he approached the responsible Board of Guardians of the local parish (St James) and successfully persuaded them to remove the handle of the pump. The outbreak immediately began to subside.

In spite of the apparent success of this manoeuvre a degree of official scepticism persisted. The Board of Health itself, having had access to all the relevant data, was difficult to convince:

> *In explanation of the remarkable intensity of this outbreak within very definite limits, it has been suggested by Dr Snow that the real cause of whatever was peculiar in the case lay in the general use of one particular well, situate at Broad Street in the middle of the district, and having (it was imagined) its waters contaminated by the rice water evacuations of cholera patients. After careful inquiry we see no reason to adopt this belief* (General Board of Health 1854).

And, in fact, there *were* certain aspects of the matter which at first did appear at variance with Dr Snow's conclusions. A widow and her niece, living in Hampstead and Islington respectively, died at the same time as the Soho epidemic was raging. However Dr Snow, pursuing his quest relentlessly, visited the widow's son and found that his mother had considered the water from the Broad Street pump particularly palatable and had had a large bottle of it delivered to her home by cart daily. Both she and her niece had "enjoyed" this water at the very start of the Soho epidemic. Yet again, there was a brewery in Broad Street itself employing 70 local workers, none of whom had become victims of the disease. However Snow readily found the explanation of this anomaly: these employees were given a free allowance of beer every day and so were not in the habit of drinking any water at all! (Summers 1989).

Still determined to prove his case beyond reasonable doubt Dr Snow pressed on to find further situations which, he hoped, would demonstrate the inevitable logic of his conclusions. He did not have long to wait as he realised that the pattern of distribution of a part of London's water supply would readily provide him with the material for a comparative study.

He was able to show that households obtaining their water supply from the Southwark and Vauxhall Company were much more likely to succumb to cholera than those drinking water from the Lambeth Company. Given that he had already established that the former company's source was a polluted stretch of the Thames and that the latter extracted its water from much further upstream, clear of the effluents further downstream, he already had what might be regarded as *prima facie* evidence of cause and effect. What made the comparison even more conclusive was the fact that, in situations where adjacent houses were supplied by the two different companies, a "Southwark and Vauxhall" house was 14 times more likely to suffer a cholera death than a house supplied by the Lambeth Company (Adler 2004). It would indeed be difficult for a miasma to operate in such a manner!

Dr Snow included these additional findings in a second report, also entitled *On the Mode of Communication of Cholera* (1855), demonstrating clearly that cholera infection could not only be carried in water but also spread by contaminated food and transmitted from to person through soiling of hands (Longmate 1966). But, although Pelling (1978) expressed the view that "these demonstrations end any uncritical reign that miasmatism may have enjoyed," even Dr John Simon was among the many who still believed that contagion of the type described by Dr Snow could not act without other factors being present, such as a certain state of the atmosphere, condition of the soil etc. (Rosen 1958). The problem was, of course, that the kind of proof which might have convinced the sceptics was still lacking, and would not in fact be available until 1884 when Dr Robert Koch, a young German microbiologist was able to demonstrate the existence of the cholera microbe, the *Vibrio Cholerae*. And indeed the evolution of what was to become the study of animal and human microbiology was already taking place on the European Continent and Koch's demonstration of the cholera germ was simply one discovery in a sequence which had begun half a century earlier in Italy.

It is a commonplace experience that certain actions can lead to unexpected outcomes further along the line—the so-called "law of unintended consequences." And so it was with the laboratory demonstration of forms of microbial life which might be responsible for disease. The earliest evidence emerged from the world of the silk industry in Lombardy. Agostino Bassi was able to show in 1834 that muscardine, a lethal epidemic disease of silkworms, was due to a contagious living agent which subsequently turned out to be a parasitic fungus. In conjunction with his colleague Jean Victor Audouin he was able to prove that inoculating healthy silkworms with the fungus induced the disease, thereby establishing a cause-and-effect sequence under experimental conditions (Major 1944).

Subsequent to Bassi's work, a book entitled *Pathologische Untersuchungen* (Pathology Investigations) by Jacob Henle, Professor of Anatomy at Zurich, appeared in 1840, representing what we would nowadays refer to as a meta-analysis of a variety of published scientific works, including those of Bassi and Audouin, and came to the conclusion that communicable diseases were caused by living microscopic organisms. He was unable, however, to show clearly that a particular germ was responsible for a specific disease. Such proof had to await the outcome of the work of Robert Koch, one of his students some 30 years later (Rosen 1958) as is outlined below.

Curiously enough it was again concern about disease in the silkworm industry, this time in France, that provided the background to the next stage in this sequence. Dr Louis Pasteur, who in the 1860s had been originally involved in studies of fermentation of wine and beer, had come to the conclusion that this was caused by microorganisms that could be killed by heat. Thus the word "pasteurisation" entered the language, usually these days applied to milk. Not unreasonably, his work in both these fields led him to the idea that microorganisms might also infect animals and humans, thereby causing disease, but he did not find it possible to link one microbe with a specific infection.

Robert Koch, mentioned above, took the opportunity of developing the work of Pasteur further in the late 1870s by setting out the following rules (which subsequently became known as Koch's Postulates) for determining whether a specific living organism causes a particular disease:

1. the organism must be present in every case of the disease;
2. the organism must be able to be isolated and grown in pure culture;
3. the organism must, when inoculated into a susceptible animal, cause the specific disease;
4. the organism must then be recoverable from the animal and identified.

Anthrax was the first disease which he showed was able to meet these criteria, which then became the basis for investigating a number of further serious infectious diseases in humans (Beaglehole et al. 1993).

It will have been noted, by this point, that during the period 1830s–1870s many important developments had been taking place in not only the organisation of public health services in England but also the evolution of medical microbiology on the European Continent. These events were occurring broadly in parallel, but it is worth considering what points of contact there might have been and more specifically to what extent English public health thinking and legislation were being informed by the findings from the various Continental laboratories. It is perhaps simplistic to imagine that a discovery at location X will soon modify practice at location Y. There are already well-understood criteria for testing the various processes and effects of a communication of this sort: were the facts adequately known beyond location X? Were they understood, given that different languages might be involved (e.g. Henle's *Pathologische Untersuchungen*)? Were they convincing enough to cause reappraisal of existing ideas? Lastly, did they actually modify professional practice? It is worth examining these points in a little detail.

It would be easy to imagine that England, with its traditional cultural insularity, might have been relatively unaware of significant developments on the Continent. This however was not totally the case, in this instance at least. John Simon, who was probably regarded as the "market leader" in English public health thinking at this time, was far from insular in his outlook. As a young man he had travelled widely in Europe, taking note of the public health systems of the various countries, and meeting key figures such as Jacob Henle, although as late as the 1840s and early 1850s he dismissed the latter's germ theory as unproven, considering the phenomena of infective diseases to be essentially chemical (Simon 1850). And even although Henle's germ theory, explicitly set out in *Pathologische Untersuchungen* in 1840, was supported by the empirical observations of John Snow, it gained little credence in England generally, during this period. Even Pasteur's demonstration, during the early 1860s, of the existence of pathogenic organisms was slow in having an effect and as late as 1869–1872 some distinguished Medical Officers of Health could still attribute diseases such as typhoid to "the insidious miasm" of sewer gases and dismiss germs as "nothing but nonsense" (National Association for the Promotion of Social Science 1869).

By the mid-1870s, however, the old "atmospheric" views of the 1850s and the compromise position of the 1860s had been given up in the light of new discoveries and "*Simon could finally and excitedly accept specific contagion as the cause of infection*" (Lambert 1963). However, as Porter (1999) has pointed out, Simon was convinced that more than simply infection was responsible for the occurrence of disease, and that the health of the community was governed by social, economic and political factors with poverty representing the underlying major problem. And indeed, although this piece of work is focused specifically on the epidemiological and microbiological aspects of the control of communicable diseases, it is obvious that the "germ theory" could not ever represent the complete picture; a combination of genetic, immunological, nutritional and socio-economic factors may also play a part. [McKeown (1979) has particularly stressed the specific importance of nutrition and housing in this realm]. For example, by no means everyone exposed to the organisms of tuberculosis, poliomyelitis or meningococcal infection will necessarily develop clinical evidence of disease.

And so it can be seen that the impact of cholera, (the title of this chapter), in the most positive sense, was that its invasion of England in 1831 signalled the need for local public health action within the country, resulting in the setting up of **a network of authorities which was to become England's first nation-wide system of public health**. At the same time, but starting from a quite different base, Chadwick's idea of **a "public doctor" to have formal responsibility to the local community for, *inter alia*, the control of infectious diseases resulted in the concept of the Medical Officer of Health**, an office which was to last for well over a century, taking on additional responsibilities or transferring others in response to a variety of factors ranging from national social conscience, through war and its aftermath to major political and organizational change. While the office lasted, however, it never relinquished its basic responsibility for the prevention and control of communicable diseases at local level (supported by many new findings in the expanding field of bacteriology), until the post itself was abolished by the reorganization of the National Health Service and local government in 1974, when alternative arrangements were made; these are dealt with as appropriate in subsequent chapters.

Addendum

The period of a 100 years or so from the establishment of the office of Medical Officer of Health until its demise in the latter part of the twentieth century probably represents the most exhaustively documented era in English public health history and therefore there is no intention in this work to go over this ground in detail once more. Accordingly the following brief commentary does no more than attempt to bridge the gap between the developments outlined in the first three chapters and the real "meat" of the book, which is primarily concerned with events from the run up to the Second World War onwards.

Although, as was stated earlier, the permissive powers of the 1848 Public Health Act allowed the appointment of Medical Officers of Health, not every town and by no means every rural district created such a post at that point. The 1872 Act theoretically made such appointments compulsory but, even by the following year, in practice such posts were simply deemed advisable (Frazer 1950). In fact, Coventry City Council appeared to have been rather complacent when it appointed Dr Mark Anthony Fenton MD in 1874, stating (in his obituary in *The Times* of 6th April 1897) that "The Council were wise in taking time by the forelock as, under the 1875 Act, such posts were to be truly mandatory."

It seems that, in making this appointment, Coventry City Council had indeed been fortunate as Dr Fenton was a cultured and professionally distinguished member of the medical profession. An Arts graduate of Trinity College Dublin, he had gone on to qualify first in surgery, then in midwifery and finally in medicine itself in 1870. Three years later he had obtained the degree of Doctor of Medicine (MD), then as now a *higher* medical qualification indicating both excellence and proof of having made an original contribution to the sum of medical scientific knowledge. The particular relevance of this higher qualification was that Dr Fenton had acquired it before the Medical Act of 1886 made a higher, specialized qualification a formal requirement for the holding of a post of this sort. In this respect he would appear to have satisfied one of the most important criteria laid down by Chadwick in his Report to Poor Law Commissioners regarding his recommended position of "district medical officer." Furthermore, as was pointed out in his obituary in *The Herald* dated 9th April 1897, among Medical Officers of Health in the Midlands, Dr Fenton had held a high position and was at one time President of the Birmingham Medical Association.

It will have been noted that the Medical Officer of Health post came into being, almost by chance, alongside major engineering developments which were essentially intended to provide pure water supplies and a more effective means of removing human and other waste. As is pointed out below, such technical advances were more likely to have a beneficial effect on the incidence of communicable diseases spread by water, foodstuffs or physical contact with insanitary materials than on infectious diseases spread e.g. by droplet spray from the nose or mouth.

If the Medical Officer of Health were to be able to make any impact on the febrile conditions in his District he clearly first needed to have details of the relevant cases, and ideally having the first case reported to him, to alert him. Although the statistics provided by the arrangement initiated by enthusiasts from the like of John Graunt through to William Farr gave a general picture of the pattern of disease, what the Medical Officer of Health required is what we would nowadays refer to as "real time" data re individual cases as they were actually occurring, in other words a surveillance system based on some kind of formal case reporting. Although as far back as the 1860s John Simon had been calling for an effective system of notification of cases so that they could be isolated, it was not until 1889 that this became a legal requirement and, at that stage, only as far as London was concerned (Holland and Stewart 1997). The frustration caused by the lack of such a system is clearly shown in the 1882 Annual Report of the Medical Officer of Health of Coventry, in which, speaking of smallpox in the City, Dr Fenton stated:

> *From the experience gained in Coventry of late years, I do not consider that there should ever be any difficulty in preventing smallpox from assuming any serious proportions* ***if only the medical profession and the public will assist by giving immediate information of the first outbreak*** (Fenton 1882).

The 1889 Infectious Disease (Notification) Act listed smallpox, cholera, diphtheria, membranous croup, erysipelas, scarlatina (scarlet fever) and any of the fevers known as typhus, typhoid, enteric, relapsing, continued or puerperal as diseases which required to be notified primarily by the head of the family but more significantly, as far as clinical details were concerned, by the medical practitioner attending the case. It was not until 10 years later, in 1899, that such provisions were extended to cover the whole of England. Fortunately for Coventry, "*through Dr Fenton's instrumentality a system of inter-notification of cases of infectious diseases in and around the City was established in 1895, as a result of which many a serious epidemic has been averted*" (Obituary in *The Herald* dated 9th April 1897). It is interesting to note that such inter-authority cooperation was still not uniformly applicable between the 41 District Health Authorities across Greater London as recently as 1993 (Pollock 1993).

Although the major piece of consolidating public health legislation—the 1875 Public Health Act—had included among the duties of the Medical Officer of Health "the suppression of diseases," those newly appointed to such posts clearly had to consider just exactly what they could actually do, in practice, to control outbreaks of infectious disease in their Districts. Apart from vaccination against smallpox, theoretically the measures could only be those which had applied from the Middle Ages—isolation of patients, quarantine of contacts, and general sanitary measures. The sanitary reformers were firmly of the belief that efficient measures of general sanitation would be sufficient in controlling all of them. However as the second half of the century gradually shed light on the nature of the organisms causing specific diseases it became clear that such measures had a greater potential to reduce the incidence of diseases such as cholera, typhoid and dysentery than droplet-borne infections such as smallpox, diphtheria and scarlatina (Frazer 1950). (Interestingly, however, Jefferson et al. (2009) have been among the more recent workers to show that handwashing and other measures of *personal* hygiene can also contribute significantly to the reduction of spread of *respiratory* viruses, in addition to infections usually spread by the faecal-oral route.)

As has been mentioned in the last paragraph of Chap. 3, Medical Officers of Health were, over a period, required to take on many other public health responsibilities, i.e. additional to working with others in the attempt to secure a hygienic environment, and being personally responsible for preventing and controlling infectious diseases in their Districts. As the late nineteenth century rolled forwards to the twentieth, social concerns led to the idea of development of personal health services, initially focusing on mothers and children. For example in 1902 an Act established a central register of midwives which guaranteed appropriate standards for the management of childbirth. Purely fortuitously, within 2 years, as a result of a report which showed that very many young men recruited to fight in the Boer War were in an extremely poor state of health, the Government brought in a system of medical inspection of schoolchildren (essentially viewed as potential army recruits). Thus it can be seen that a rudimentary form of personal health care system was being brought in which, however limited, theoretically covered the period from before birth to school-leaving age.

The end of the First World War resulted in a further demand for the development of health care services for mothers and children, resulting in the passing of the Maternity and Child Welfare Act of 1918 which required local authorities "to attend to the health of expectant and nursing mothers and of children under 5 years of age not yet at school." It appeared to make sense that the local authority's Medical Officer of Health should be asked to organize such services and the post then became known as Medical Officer of Health and School Medical Officer.

Many other personal health services—for the aged, the mentally deficient and lunatics (to quote the thoughtlessly unkind terminology of the period!) were tacked on to the Medical Officer of Health's department, only to be subsequently redistributed appropriately to other institutions as hospitals and local authority social welfare services were developed. Apart from two groups, namely those suffering from tuberculosis or venereal diseases, the above services are not relevant to the scope of this book which, it is hoped, is demonstrating a continuing "thread" of the arrangements in England for the control of communicable diseases.

Chapter 4
Stiffening the Sinews

In peace there's nothing so becomes a man
As modest stillness and humility:
But when the blast of war blows in our ears,
Then imitate the action of the tiger;
Stiffen the sinews, summon up the blood

(William Shakespeare, *The Life of King Henry V*, Act 3 Scene 1)

The origin of the concept of the post of Medical Officer of Health has been dealt with in detail in the previous chapter. The first time I personally came across a real live example of such an individual coincided with my having to confront the reality that the onset of the Second World War was imminent. It was August 1939, I was 9 years old and I was being medically examined by Dr Harry Rae, the well-known Medical Officer of Health of the City of Aberdeen, in order to obtain an FFI (Freedom from Infection) Certificate prior to being evacuated forthwith to the United States to live with my father's aunt in Buffalo, New York State. The FFI examination was a rather cursory affair, searching for skin infections, scalp infestation etc. and the chest was auscultated. An additional embarrassment was the inclusion of a brief test for hernia. When Dr Rae said "Cough" I thought he was asking a question and replied in the negative, earning a sharp prod from my mother! It was 17 years before I saw Dr Rae again, this time as a visiting lecturer on my postgraduate course at Aberdeen University. (This early encounter was to have a profound impact on my own subsequent career in public health, as the image with which I was confronted was that of a white-coated, stethoscope-wielding *clinician*, carrying out medical examinations on individuals just like any family doctor or hospital specialist. This professional role model was the one I instinctively adopted in due course, as I moved through the grades of the public health service, retaining personal clinical responsibility at all times for infectious disease control, even alongside my formal management responsibilities as head of department, until I retired. To have given up this particular branch of clinical work completely would, for me, have removed a major part of the satisfaction of being a public health doctor.)

G. Pollock, *An Epidemiological Odyssey: The Evolution of Communicable Disease Control*, DOI 10.1007/978-94-007-3998-7_4,

Most of my classmates were headed for Canada, which had offered to take large groups of British children and find appropriate homes for them, but I was fortunate in that I was going to the home of a family member whom I had met and liked a great deal. I must admit that, in a childish way, I rather enjoyed the special status which this gave me among my friends. America, to us at that time, meant cowboys and Indians, sky-scrapers and film stars; the cinema did not tend to portray the country's heavy industry! In any event I never did get to Buffalo, by reason of an act of war referred to below.

But, as far back as early 1938, the British Government had already been alive to the possibility of war. About 18 months before all the children described above were being "processed" for immediate evacuation abroad (the arrangements for which were aborted at a stroke because of the sinking of the British liner *Athenia* by a German submarine on the second day of the war) the Government had already been taking steps to plan for an emergency service which would assist in dealing with the risk of serious epidemics arising from a number of factors such as the likely large movements of both civilian population and the Armed Forces, crowding in air raid shelters, the possibility that the enemy might adopt bacteriological warfare, and the expectation that bombing could damage both sewers and water mains.

The risk of war causing epidemics had, in fact, drawn to the Government's attention the fact that there was a considerable irregularity in the distribution of public health laboratories in the country. Writing in 1946, reviewing the state of the public health during the war years, the Chief Medical Officer of the Ministry of Health stated simply "Before the war no public health laboratory service existed for the country as a whole" (Ministry of Health 1946). Local authorities themselves were at that time responsible for the provision of laboratory support to their Medical Officer of Health in the discharge of his duties for the prevention and control of infectious diseases, a form of assistance the need for which had been identified originally by Sir John Simon (Frazer 1950). However, as Wilson (1951) pointed out, as laboratory reporting on each specimen meant a bill being sent to the local authority, this resulted in small outbreaks being neglected and even larger outbreaks tending to be investigated in a hasty and superficial manner.

Landsborough Thomson (1943) has explained how the new service was set up and organised. The preparations, begun early in 1938, included entrusting the planning and direction of the proposed service—the Emergency Public Health Laboratory Service (EPHLS)—to the Medical Research Council, acting on behalf of the Ministry of Health. The main service covered England and Wales, excluding the metropolitan area, Greater London having its own arrangements. Existing laboratories in universities, schools and other institutions were identified in advance and earmarked for this future role, and bacteriologists normally engaged in teaching and research joined with those of the Ministry of Health's own laboratory to be ready to staff the new service. These arrangements allowed the EPHLS to be mobilised immediately on the outbreak of war. The Service consisted initially of central laboratories in Oxford, Cambridge and Cardiff, along with a number of smaller laboratories throughout England and Wales. The understanding was that the Emergency Laboratories would be asked to undertake all the work of the local authorities in their area in return for a contributory payment based on peacetime expenditure.

It is perhaps worthwhile taking a quick look at the general epidemiological situation which prevailed in the country at the time when the EPHLS was moving into operation. The Ministry of Health records for the year 1938 highlighted the following matters of interest:

Deaths from **tuberculosis** represented the lowest ever recorded: 26,176 compared with 28,529 in the previous year and 35,818 in 1931.

The outlook with regard to **diphtheria** was stated to be "disappointing:" 65,008 notifications with a case fatality rate of 4.5%, compared with 61,341 in the previous year and 57,785 in 1936. The Chief Medical Officer pointed out that this was the principal cause of mortality among children of school age, He emphasised that these figures need not be so high: "*Yet, for this serious disease of childhood an effective method of immunisation is available and with willing cooperation of the public an immense reduction in the incidence and number of deaths could be secured*"

(This matter is dealt with in greater detail below.)

The incidence of **acute poliomyelitis**, 1,489 cases with 172 deaths, represented a peak year since notification became compulsory in 1912.

Cerebro-spinal fever continued to increase: 1,288 cases with 652 deaths. The point was made that with early admission to hospital and use of sulphonamides the case fatality rate might be cut to about 4%.

The year produced 18 cases of **smallpox**, all of which were infected outside England.

Comment was made on the considerable decline in the incidence of the **enteric group of fevers** since the latter years of the nineteenth century, as a result of the purification of water supplies, the pasteurisation of milk, hygienic food practices and the control of "carriers."

Figures from the Venereal Disease Treatment Centres showed that the incidence of both **syphilis** and **gonorrhoea** was declining, in the latter instance at least in part due to treatment by sulphonamides (Ministry of Health 1938).

Banks (1948) has drawn attention to the fact that, in spite of the anxieties concerning the public health felt by the Government at the beginning of the war, the country did not, in fact, experience large-scale epidemics or bacteriological warfare. As a consequence the EPHLS quickly developed along other lines. Initially Medical Officers of Health tended to use the laboratories simply for the examination of individual specimens, but quite soon it became obvious that there was an opportunity for team work in tackling outbreaks of infectious disease, with cooperation between the Medical Officer of Health, the director of the laboratory, the general practitioners and the regional medical officers of the Ministry of Health. Additionally an information service was rapidly developed whereby news of any unusual incidence of infectious disease was immediately notified to the regional office, along with any unusual or suspicious laboratory finding, resulting in a weekly infectious diseases bulletin being circulated to each Medical Officer of Health. Fortunately the EPHLS was able to persuade local authorities that, on the basis of an appropriate financial arrangement, their Medical Officers of Health could have unlimited service within an agreed schedule of the tests required for the control of infectious disease in the community (Williams 1987). This rapidly became highly relevant as outbreaks of diphtheria started to occur in village schools consequent upon the coming together of town and country children which resulted from evacuation. Medical Officers of Health, tied up in administrative duties, had no spare time for the proper investigation of these outbreaks, and many were only too ready to delegate this task to the new laboratories (Wilson 1951).

Right from the beginning, however, it was made clear that such fieldwork was to be undertaken by the laboratories only at the request of, or with the consent of, the Medical Officer of Health, in whom alone the final responsibility was vested and on whom statutory obligations were laid. The function of the laboratory was to provide him with all the information which a modern laboratory was capable of giving him and to offer advice, if appropriate, on how this information might be used to control any specific outbreak (Ministry of Health 1946). From the above account one could detect a certain tentativeness in the arrangements, as the EPHLS clearly did not wish to appear to be intruding on the professional "territory" of the Medical Officer of Health, a situation which in a sense could be regarded as a microcosm of the interface between Central and Local Government. [Even as late as the 1990s this situation was one which had to be handled with professional delicacy (Pollock 1993) as is illustrated in Chap. 7 concerning events in Greater London.] On the positive side however, the arrangements were greatly welcomed as a Medical Officer of Health could now take advantage of the availability of considerable expertise in bacteriology and immunology without having to be concerned about the cost of any operation in the field. For example, writing in his Annual Report for the years 1939–1945, the Chief Medical Officer stated: "*In the control of diphtheria a method comprising active and passive immunisation of the children exposed to risk, together with the temporary segregation of carriers, proved so reliable that outbreaks were brought to an abrupt end without closing the school or institution for even a day*" (Ministry of Health 1946). Additionally the benefits of having an integrated microbiology service were demonstrated, for example by having been able to unravel a number of small outbreaks of typhoid as a result of applying a phage-typing system, and also having the facility to identify salmonella types, thereby demonstrating, for instance, that particular outbreaks of food-poisoning had been caused by dried egg imported from the United States (Williams 1987).

The paradox was that, not only was there no attempt on the part of the Germans to employ bacteriological warfare, the incidence of infectious diseases in England during the war years was in fact remarkably low, with no serious epidemics except one of cerebro-spinal fever, and an increase in epidemic hepatitis in both troops and civilians. Influenza had been greatly feared but in the six winters, three of which were severe, only two brief epidemics of mild disease occurred. Twenty-seven cases of smallpox were notified, 16 acquired abroad and the remaining 11 secondary to one of them. In 1943 "infective jaundice" was made compulsorily notifiable in East Anglia to allow the Medical Research Council staff to attempt to discriminate between the infectious condition and "serum jaundice" following injection of a therapeutic substance (McNalty 1953). East Anglia would appear to have been a particularly suitable area for this research as it was a designated "reception area," accepting around 240,000 "official" evacuees (mothers and children and the infirm), along with many more "unofficial" ones arriving by private arrangement, within the first few months of the outbreak of war (Banks 1948). Water-borne disease, in spite of earlier fears, did not become a reality. In the summer of 1940, in order to prevent intentional pollution by enemy agents, the Ministry of Health formally required chlorination of main water supplies. Similarly, actions by the Ministry and the various local authorities were successful in preventing contamination of water supplies even when, during the air raids of 1940/1941, many water mains were fractured and sewage mains also suffered damage.

Sociologists and social psychologists are no doubt familiar with the phenomenon by which a group of people who are brought together for a specific purpose may continue to meet together on an on-going basis for professional (or even social) reasons long after the original purpose has ceased to apply. The creation of the EPHLS had brought together from different parts of the country key individuals with shared professional interests, some of whom had never even met the others previously. The novelty and value of this large coordinated group must have been extremely stimulating to all its members. Williams (1985) relates how the war-time service had soon established a strong *esprit de corps* with staff having a great respect for the liberal administrative traditions of the Medical Research Council. If, as was widely believed, the Ministry of Health had possibly had second thoughts on financial grounds about bringing such a service into being, given that the dangers which had caused their anxieties had not materialised, it was almost certainly too late; the genie was out of the bottle and was not going to go back in!

When the service was reviewed after 3 or 4 years of operation there was no doubt that it had been remarkably successful. The Chief Medical Officer of the Ministry of Health, writing in 1946, went so far as to say that its discontinuance at the end of the war would have been unthinkable (Ministry of Health 1946). And so, when in 1945 the Government decided to retain the service on a permanent footing, the Medical Research Council agreed to run it for a further 5 years. In due course, however, the service had established such a distinct identity for itself that all were agreed that it should be administered by its own Public Health Laboratory Service Board acting as an agent of the Ministry of Health, and this was indeed achieved by the Public Health Laboratory Service Act 1960.

Another key development at this time was the introduction of diphtheria immunisation (known colloquially at the time as “inoculation”) which, along with smallpox vaccination, was to form the core of routine childhood protection in England. Although work on what were to become passive and active protection against diphtheria had been initiated in France and Germany towards the end of the nineteenth century and active immunisation of New York City schoolchildren had begun in 1921 (Hammonds 1993) the procedure was relatively late to arrive in England. This was not because the Ministry of Health itself was unaware of the possibilities. In 1922 it had issued a Memorandum on methods of active immunisation against the disease, followed by a more detailed document, *The Production of Artificial Immunity against Diphtheria*, in 1932. The Chief Medical Officer expressed his disappointment at this situation when he stated “*Artificial immunisation against diphtheria continues to make progress but slowly. Its value is undeniable and is as yet not sufficiently appreciated, nor is the toll of death which diphtheria exacts among the child population*." The view has been expressed that during the 1920s and 1930s, by which time effective immunisation agents were available in England, Medical Officers of Health had become too involved in day-to-day administrative duties, particularly in respect of municipal hospitals, to exploit this new preventive measure. In any event this would have required a measure of determination in the difficult financial circumstances of the 1930s (Lewis 1991).

Consideration needs to be given, however, to other possible reasons for the delay in offering this valuable protection against this principal killing disease of school-age children, especially when there were no specific remedies against the *other* childhood infections spread by droplet spray, e.g. scarlet fever, measles or whooping-cough, diseases also with significant mortality. Newman (1933) had pointed out how the control of such "personal contact" diseases had lagged behind that of the so-called environmental diseases such as cholera and typhoid. Additionally it has to be recalled that, short of immunisation, the only measures which the Medical Officer of Health could employ to attempt to prevent the spread of diphtheria were notification, isolation in hospital and disinfection (i.e. little more effective than in mediaeval times). Could characteristic English "insularity" have been a relevant factor, simply ignoring what was being achieved in other parts of the world? For example in England and Wales with a population of 41 million in 1937 the incidence of diphtheria was 149 per 100,000 population. In Canada with a population of 11 million, and an active immunisation programme, the comparable rate was less than one! (Ministry of Health 1946) Perhaps a contributory factor could also have been, as Frazer (1950) suggests, that parents themselves, possibly mindful of smallpox vaccination, were disinclined to seek or accept, on behalf of their children, any method of protection which involved "penetration of the skin in some measure, however small." This last point emphasises the importance of the potential impact of the words used, the term "immunisation" almost certainly being less anxiety-provoking than "vaccination" (a lesson I learned early in my public health career).

The war had clearly brought a new dimension into this unsatisfactory situation. The risk of diphtheria epidemics as a result of children being evacuated from towns, where the disease tended to be endemic, to rural areas, where it was relatively rare, required determined action by the Government. A seven-page Ministry of Health updating document explaining the basis of both acquired and artificial immunity and making a firm set of practical recommendations—*Memorandum on the Production of Artificial Immunity against Diphtheria*—was issued in 1940. This provided the background to the beginning of a major national campaign in which the Ministry made it clear to local authorities that the antigens were to be provided free, thereby ending the prospect of the cost being borne by local ratepayers.

My recollection of being a personal recipient of this protective measure is vivid. Our first indication of anything unusual was that, as a class of 10-year olds in an East End school, we were shepherded without explanation to the "medical room," told to roll up our sleeves and stand in line, and then watched in horror as a rather brusque white-coated individual walked down the line, injecting us one after another without a pause nor a reassuring word. Standing there awaiting one's turn was unpleasant as we could see the expressions of agony on the faces of those ahead of us. One poor girl with matchstick arms shrieked as the needle clearly struck bone and her language was highly colourful. I thought I carried it off quite well although I felt rather weak at the knees and on returning to the classroom the teacher told me rather sharply that I was white as a sheet and should sit down. In wartime 1940, apparently, there was no time to treat children with kid gloves.

Presumably our parents had been consulted and had given consent but this raises an interesting point as the law with regard to compulsory vaccination was still theoretically in place (and was not finally withdrawn until 1946) but in practice the unpopularity of any kind of compulsion in personal spheres of this kind meant that the law had played a diminishing role. It is interesting to speculate whether, had the law on compulsion *been* applied, there would have been public protests similar to those of a 100 years previously in connection with smallpox vaccination. It is extremely doubtful; the mood of the country was subdued and compliant at that stage of the war, with cities being bombed, air raid precautions including blackout enforced, children evacuated, food and clothes rationed and gas-masks, sandbags and identity cards issued. Diphtheria inoculation would probably have been seen simply as yet another formal decree of the Government to protect the nation. Additionally, many adults at that time would have been able to think of at least one relation who had suffered from the disease and possibly died. I was personally aware, even at that age, that a younger sister of my mother had been fatally affected as a 2-year old. In any event the Government took the view that the responsibility for securing the protection of the individual child rested firmly with the parents, rather than with the local authority. In the words of the Chief Medical Officer, "*It is to the public that we must look for any improvement in the situation. Without their cordial cooperation it is not possible to advance.*"

The health publicity at the time gave birth to such now-familiar phrases as "*Coughs and Sneezes Spread Diseases*" but diphtheria was singled out for special attention, initially focussing on schoolchildren as a readily available "captive" population, thereafter the under-fives, and lastly infants before their first birthday. This on-going campaign represented a successful partnership between the Ministry of Health and the Ministry of Information, with the Central Council for Health Education being recognised as the responsible body for assisting local authorities in this work. Posters, leaflets, and radio talks by the Chief Medical Officer personally were supplemented by advertisements in both national and local newspapers, all encouraging parents to have their children immunised.

In Coventry, when immunisation was introduced in 1941, 4,376 children received the procedure, the majority at school. In the Annual Report of the Medical Officer of Health and School Medical Officer, Dr (later Sir Alfred) A Massey wrote:

> *It is again emphasised that diphtheria is still a menace to child life and health and parents should regard it as a primary duty to their children to have them immunised against the disease. There are full facilities for this in the schools. At the year-end the local campaign was gaining momentum* (Massey 1941).

There appeared to be little or no public debate about the matter, certainly no evidence of parental opposition. Trawling through all the issues of the local newspaper, *The Coventry Standard*, for that year revealed only two mentions of the topic, the first in a report of an address of a strongly supportive nature to the Coventry Rotary Club by a local general practitioner, Dr D Murray Bladon, and the second, a letter from a Miss L Loat, Secretary of the National Anti-Vaccination League, challenging Dr Bladon's views on all immunisation and vaccination procedures. In fact, in the Coventry of 1941 as portrayed in the local press, the word immunisation tended to be used more in connection with protection against typhoid fever as the intense air raids had caused widespread damage to both public water supplies and drainage, and Dr Massey had arranged for the provision of facilities for immunisation against this disease, along with advising that drinking water should be boiled.

The national immunisation scheme was finally fully implemented by the end of 1941. The impact was impressive, mortality from the disease falling by one-third within a year and by three-quarters by 1946. Holland and Stewart (1997) have estimated, however, that failing to introduce the procedure during the 1930s, when it would have been feasible, probably resulted in 20,000 avoidable deaths from the disease during that decade. An *Enquiry* carried out by *The Social Survey* for the Ministry of Health at the end of the war showed that 67% of children under the age of 16, approximately 50% of those under 5, and about 20% of infants less than 2 years of age had been immunised. There were no significant differences between rural and urban districts but the proportion immunised was lower in the North of England—59% compared with around 70% in the other regions. On being asked the question "Do you know how diphtheria can be prevented?" 78% of mothers had mentioned immunisation. It was surprising, therefore, that only 24% knew that it was an infectious disease, many others thinking that it was due to drains or dirt, or simply admitted to not knowing. On the topic of publicity, 87% had seen the posters, 75% had read about the subject in newspapers and magazines, 50% had heard about it on the radio and 40% had noticed the cinema publicity. Reasons given for children *not* being immunised ranged from mothers stating that they simply had not had the time or had "not bothered" (23%) to mothers expressing the belief that it was not necessary or might hurt or frighten their child, or that their husband objected (26%). In between, lay a miscellany of replies which could not be classified as apathy or resistance e.g. the child would soon be immunised, had already had diphtheria or was too young etc., responses the validity of which were more difficult to assess. Fortunately only 1% of mothers with immunised children had experienced any difficulty in getting the procedure carried out (Box 1945).

War has, of course, a tendency to disrupt stable social structures and conventional behaviour. Reference has been made above to the population movements including evacuation of mothers and children from cities to the countryside, but also relevant factors were conscription of young men and women into the Armed Forces and a variety of other personnel engaged in essential war work, almost by definition representing the younger half of the age spectrum, displaced and living in unfamiliar surroundings. One has also to consider the anxieties and heightened tensions felt by many individuals removed, not by choice, from their usual reassuring contact with family members and friends. On the other hand war can be exciting, especially for young people, and there can be little doubt that many young adults found the experience not unpleasurable. Some, especially young women, may have found relief from the tedium of an unrewarding repetitive job, or even from oppressive family circumstances including constant vigilance by—in their view—over-concerned parents. Furthermore the possibility of making new friends would be of interest to those with a more outgoing personality. (An aunt of mine, my mother's youngest sister, for example, readily relinquished a boring office job, enlisted in the Women's Branch of the Royal Air Force and happily drove a three-ton truck for the duration of the war, meeting her future husband in the Services.) Certainly many wartime novels and films have a central theme of romantic and passionate relationships, tinged with the unsettling emotions of being parted.

Consequently in 1938 the Government, mindful of the threat of war, assumed that the situation described above would probably lead to a degree of loosening of the usual self-control which tends to govern social behaviour in the stable conditions of peacetime. Additionally there was an acknowledgement of the fact that, with a sudden increase in the population of rural areas, sexual promiscuity might lead to an increase in the incidence of venereal diseases in localities poorly provided with facilities for the treatment of these conditions.

Accordingly, writing in his 1938 Annual Report on the State of the Public Health, the Chief Medical Officer considered that it would be necessary for county councils and county boroughs in some areas to expand existing centres and in others to set up additional ones to cope with outbreaks in places from which infected persons could not attend existing facilities. As at that time it was impossible to determine where the greatest pressure on services might occur he felt that the best approach would be to form mobile units each consisting of a specialist in venereal diseases, a nurse, an orderly and a clerk, with a motor vehicle containing all necessary equipment to enable these diseases to be treated efficiently. Such units could also take over the work of any existing centre which had been depleted of personnel removed for other wartime duties (Ministry of Health 1938).

In fact, during the Second World War, social disruption was much greater than could have been envisaged in 1938. In addition to the population movements already referred to, the country found itself having to accommodate members of the Armed Forces of many other nations who joined with the indigenous ones in training activities, air operations against the enemy and ultimately the planned invasion of Europe in 1944. It was assumed, therefore, that sexual promiscuity on an even greater scale would be an inevitable consequence and that venereal diseases would be, even more than usually, "the camp follower of war."

The Government's reaction was to look to health education as a primary means of prevention and control. This was not a totally new approach to the problem.

Fraser Brockington (1966) describes how the British Social Hygiene Council was formed for this purpose in 1915 from an amalgamation of so-called "Abolitionist Associations," and how a decade later local authorities were given powers to put such health education on a more formal basis. Interestingly he concludes that from that point "the taboo was off and enlightenment began." He was perhaps somewhat optimistic in this judgment. As late as 1986, in my capacity of District Medical Officer for Coventry, I encountered considered resistance from the editor of the local newspaper when I expressed a wish to write a feature explaining the facts concerning HIV infection. His attitude—which was by no means unique—could be summed up as "We can't allow language like that, Doc, this is a *family* newspaper."

But the war was already 3 years old before the Government actually began to use public educational methods to explain the risks of venereal diseases, although these were already well established in the United States. The success of such an approach in 1940 to promote the diphtheria inoculation campaign had no doubt proved its potential although the subject matter would clearly have to be given careful consideration in order to avoid offending particular sensitivities.

In his Report on the State of the Public Health During 6 Years of War, the Chief Medical Officer made it clear that the first objective of the venereal diseases campaign was to break the "taboo" on public discussion of the problem, through the ordinary channels of publicity—the press and the radio—and employing "shock" tactics. This was to be followed up by more detailed education (Ministry of Health 1946).

The campaign was launched in October 1942 by a broadcast, followed by a press conference. The "taboo" having been broken, the larger task was now embarked upon so that the public could be made aware of the facts concerning the causation of these diseases and how they could be cured by skilled treatment at an early stage. Press advertisements such as "Ten Plain Facts about the Venereal Diseases" and films with slightly guarded titles such as "Subject for Discussion" were used to support the campaign. The reactions of different newspapers were of interest. As Bingham (2005) has pointed out, initially the Newspaper Proprietors' Association refused to publish the material until it had been made less explicit. Subsequently one popular daily refused to print even the edited version whereas its main rival was happy to discuss the problem in unusual detail. The courageous approach of the latter was the one which appealed to the majority of the public and social surveys by accredited organisations found that this information was gratefully received by many who genuinely wanted to have a better understanding of the issues.

However what most people have tended to recall were the posters. These were widely displayed on public hoardings, at railway stations, in chemists' shops, local authority offices and public toilets. [EXAMPLE] A photographic exhibition was also created for use by local authorities around the country, but this meant that one had to actually enter the relevant hall or other building being used for this purpose. That no doubt discouraged some individuals, perhaps anxious about being seen to be exhibiting what might be regarded as a prurient interest in the subject. When the exhibition came to our town, as a 13-year old schoolboy at the time I was quietly advised by an uncle (significantly, not by my parents) that it would be in my interests to pay a visit. I did so and have to confess that some of the photographs, e.g. those of patients in the late stages of syphilis, were horrifying and the strongest possible incentive to pursue the "clean living" which the Government was urging!

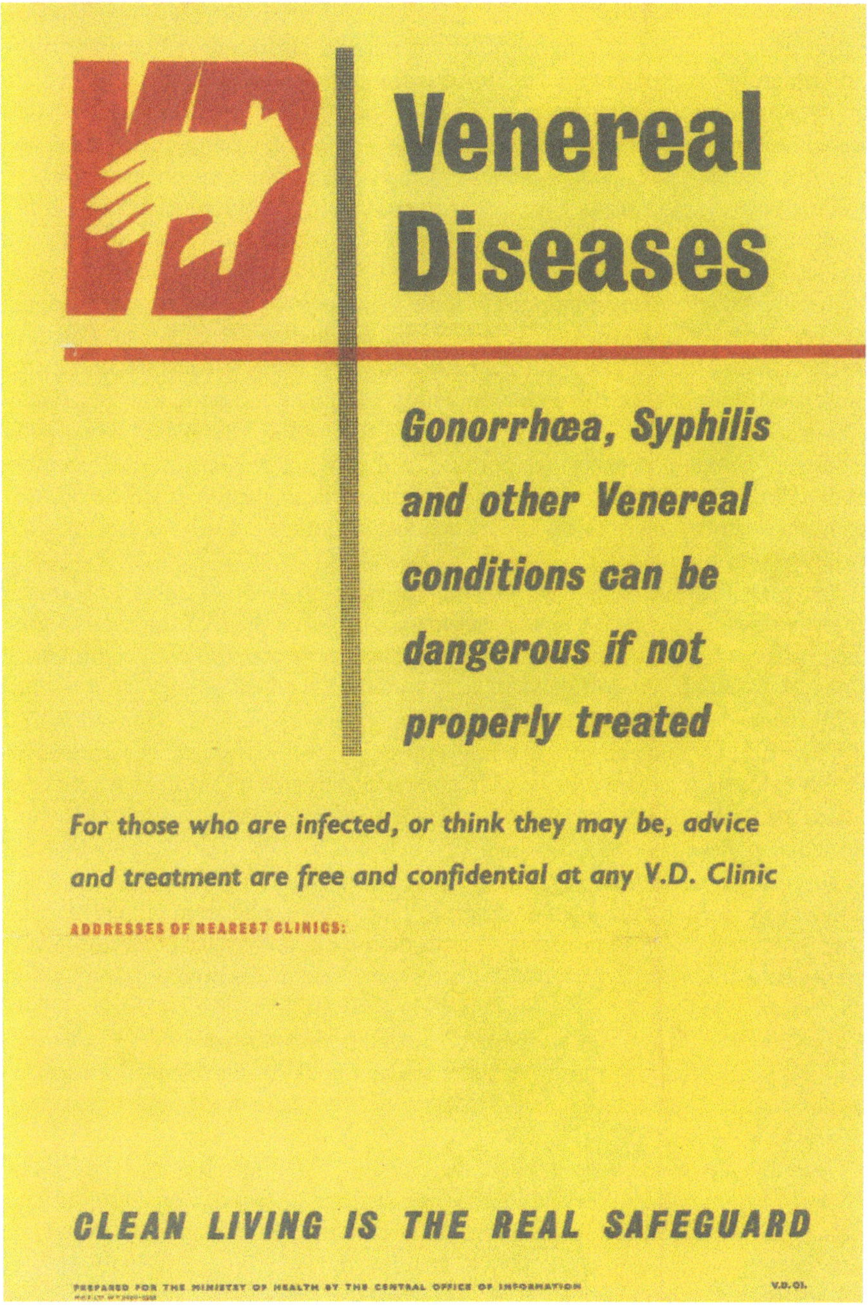

Health education messages addressed specifically to the Armed Forces had begun much earlier. A publication by Rennie Macandrew, *The Red Light*, subtitled *Intimate Hygiene for Men and Women of HM Forces*, had appeared in April 1941. Although providing a much-needed guide on sexual anatomy and physiology, it laid heavy emphasis on the dangers of venereal diseases. (Needless to say, many schoolboys managed to "borrow" copies of this publication from older brothers home on leave, and these were circulated surreptitiously in classrooms.) Lectures to the troops during basic training tended to be more graphic, and some films were quite thought-provoking. An example of the latter was that the female characters used were secretaries, typists, "respectable people"—the point being emphasised was that one couldn't tell who had VD and therefore might pass on the infection. Additionally the possible consequences of contracting VD were stated in a rather stark manner. One film showed a young man walking down to a red-light district and later wearing dark glasses because he was blind! Such films were considered of such value that the Army continued to show them to those "called up" for National Service for many years after the Second World War had ended (Hickman 2004). An arrangement of proven value was the instruction to practise self-disinfection with a prescribed pharmaceutical preparation within 10 min of exposure. This personally administered procedure had proved its value during the First World War, using potassium permanganate for this purpose, and an entry in *Hansard* on December 10th 1919 expressed the view that if only the civil population could be brought within the same framework of "instruction and discipline" as the military, they too would benefit from at least a degree of protection.

In the belief that health educational messages would not necessarily reach everyone potentially at risk or, for that matter, convince them of the need to alter their behaviour, the Government had also to consider the possibility of control measures. However society had moved a long way from the kind of legislation considered appropriate for the nineteenth century—compulsory medical examination by a naval or military surgeon of a woman believed by a special police superintendent sworn before a magistrate to be a "common prostitute," and similar attempts to police public morals (Porter 1999). Notification and compulsory treatment of syphilis had often been pressed for in the period between the two world wars but rejected as an unacceptable infringement of personal liberty. The City of Bradford in 1925 was actually able to obtain powers for the compulsory notification of venereal disease for a period of 5 years but this authorisation did not cover compulsory treatment and, as the arrangement proved relatively ineffective, the Bradford Corporation did not apply to have the powers extended beyond the 5 year period (Frazer 1950). During the Second World War, however, a compromise was adopted. On a temporary basis, syphilis was made confidentially notifiable to the Medical Officer of Health who had authority to compel treatment of any individual notified more than once (Cartwright 1977).

Additionally, social workers were recruited by VD clinics to make individuals aware of treatment facilities and to persuade contacts of cases to attend for testing. This idea, which had originated in Rotterdam in 1925 as part of the services for seamen, was in England first adopted in Tyneside in 1943. Its success there led to its being extended throughout the whole country by Regulation 33b, although the Ministry of Health's *Venereal Disease: Guide for Practitioners*, issued in 1944, made no mention of any form of social work input. Along with the successes in the use of penicillin, these determined attempts led to a considerable decrease in the incidence of syphilis so that in 1947 the formal regulations came to an end (Cartwright and Biddiss 2000). A year later, with the coming into operation of the National Health Service, the venereal disease clinics became the responsibility of the new Regional Hospital Boards, although the social workers—now known as contact tracers—remained on the staff of the Medical Officer of Health as their role was essentially of a preventive nature.

It was also during the Second World War that significant and rapid advances were made in the treatment of tuberculosis. Although a number of infectious diseases had been successfully treated by penicillin since 1941, it was not until 3 years later that an antibiotic was developed which was both active against *Mycobacterium tuberculosis* and relatively low in toxicity in test animals. On November 20 1944 this drug—*Streptomycin*—was administered for the first time to a critically ill patient. The effect was almost immediately impressive. His advanced disease was visibly arrested, the bacteria disappeared from his sputum and he made a rapid recovery (Waksman 1952). Because of the risk of drug resistance it was necessary to develop additional products which would inhibit the growth of the organism and within 10 years three further powerful drugs, PAS, INAH and *Pyrazinamide* had been added to the pharmacological armamentarium. In practice it was found that combinations of these drugs added inhibition of resistance to antibacterial activity.

Before the advent of these drugs, treatment of tuberculosis had not changed much since the sanatorium regime was introduced in the mid-nineteenth century. This form of therapy was conceived by Dr Hermann Brehmer following his personal experience of recovering from the disease as a result of undertaking restful botanical studies in the Himalayan Mountains (Kinghorn 1921). It consisted essentially of rest, good nutrition and continuous exposure to fresh air by siting beds on open balconies.

Brehmer, who was born in 1826, began to be prominent in this field in 1853 when he declared firmly that tuberculosis was a curable disease, against a background of considerable scepticism from his physician colleagues, most of whom shared the view that a diagnosis of tuberculosis represented a death sentence. Brehmer's conviction was strengthened by his awareness of the post-mortem findings of the Bohemian pathologist Rokitansky, namely that 90% of those who had not died of tuberculosis had healed tuberculous lesions within the normal lung tissue. By chance the eldest sister of Brehmer's first wife had established a small hydropathic institution in Gorbersdorf, a small village in Silesia in the midst of fir trees 715 feet above sea level and, when this did not prove commercially successful, Brehmer took it over in order to use it to prove his theories (Kinghorn 1921). Koch's discovery of the tubercle bacillus in 1882 was helpful to Brehmer's approach in that a specific cause of the disease had been identified and, of course, sanatoria provided a means by which infectious patients could be isolated from the general public. Additionally it clarified the situation which had been ill-understood: for example even such an eminent physician as Sir Thomas Watson had been satisfied that the disease did *not* spread by contagion, an assertion which he made frequently, not only at meetings of the Royal Society of Medicine but also so publicly that his views even found their way into popular medical books for the lay reader such as *Smith's Family Physician* (Smith 1873), written by the late surgeon to the emigrant ship *Amazon.*

Just before the Second World War, in the middle 1930s, artificial pneumothorax had become available in England as an adjunct to treatment for a small proportion of cases, the rationale being that a collapsed lung, or part of lung, had a better chance of healing naturally. In 1936 Dr FJ Bentley, in a Medical Research Council Special Report, reviewing the experience of using this treatment in the London County Council area, showed that in terms of lives saved there was a gain of 19.8% at the end of a 5 year period (Bentley 1936). Thoracoplasty also represented a useful form of collapse therapy for selected cases. A review of the outcome of this procedure by Gough et al. (1957) showed that, 8 years later, 82% of the patients were quiescent, 3% still had active disease, 14% had died, and 1% had been lost from the study. However 96% of the survivors traced were fit for work, all the more satisfactory as most of these patients had had extensive disease and few had received effective chemotherapy. (On the other hand, one could not deny that, from an aesthetic point of view, the physical appearance of the chest following thoracoplasty was not very much liked by many of the patients themselves.)

The Second World War might have had an impact on the services which could be provided for cases of tuberculosis as many Tuberculosis Officers had been conscripted to the Armed Forces. However in the autumn of 1939 the Minister of Health received a deputation of workers in this field and emphasis was placed on the importance of ensuring, as far as possible, that such an essential service was not put at risk by the war.

Brehmer's sanatorium concept had been copied throughout Europe and, for example, *was still in use in Britain as late as the 1950s* as a background to more active medical and/or surgical management. I can personally vouch for this in as much as in 1957 I was Resident Medical Officer at Tor-na-Dee Sanatorium situated in a fir-clad valley in North-East Scotland, where traditional rest, good nutrition and fresh air were complemented by appropriate combinations of antibiotics and, where necessary, one of a variety of thoracic surgical procedures. Tor-na-Dee was built in 1899 in the "healthy and bracing" climate of the district of Murtle as the Deeside Hydropathic. In 1918 it was converted to a 72-bedded sanatorium, originally reserved for officers and nurses returning from the First World War with tuberculosis. Treatment at that time was based on "bed rest, fresh air and contentment of mind, together with cod-liver oil, collapse of parts of the lung and graduated exercise." The establishment was ruled with a firm hand. The *Patients' Handbook* made it clear that bedroom windows had to be opened to their full extent at night, the playing of card games or draughts was allowed only with the consent of the medical staff, smoking was to be "stopped or severely rationed," and lights-out was at 10.30 pm (Culter Courier 1992—a local magazine produced by the Community Council for the district.)

The institution was one of two matching establishments together known as the Deeside Sanatoria. The other one, Glen o'Dee, was vividly portrayed by the author W Somerset Maugham (1938) in his short story *Sanatorium*, based on his personal experience of having been a patient there. The 1950 film version of the story visibly illustrated the tensions, frustrations and emotional melodramas of highly intelligent and articulate individuals confined to what seemed to them to be an indefinite period of total bed rest, with the medical attitude (meant to be soothing but sounding patronising) being summed up as "Just you lie there, and rest and time together with our regime will make you better." Fortunately from about the early 1950s the active treatment programmes, both medical and surgical, gave patients encouragement to look forward to significant clinical improvement, progressive mobilisation, and a return to normal, or near-normal, life. My own mother's bank manager, for example, was admitted to Tor-na-Dee quite seriously ill, but in due course I had the pleasure of seeing him back in his office, dealing with my mother's modest financial affairs.

However that which was beneficial for tuberculosis sufferers raised a particular problem for me regarding my own career path. In 1950, as medical students during our first term on the hospital wards, we had been told by the professor that tuberculosis in Scotland would take at least a couple of generations to deal with adequately as many patients were dying at home because of the long waiting lists for admission to hospital. Now, just 7 years later, I was finding that as a result of the dramatic effectiveness of combinations of drugs it seemed that the disease could soon be eliminated at least as a condition requiring in-patient care. This conclusion was strengthened by the senior hospital medical officer for Deeside Sanatoria, Dr Ronald Mavor, then still in his early 30s, telling me that he could not see much of a professional future for himself in this field and that he had decided to accept an invitation from the editor of *The Scotsman*, Scotland's national broadsheet, to become its drama critic and carry on his family's established literary tradition—his father was the famous Scottish playwright with the pen-name James Bridie .(In fact he went on to have a distinguished career as a playwright, Director of the Scottish Arts Council and finally Professor and Head of the Department of Drama at Saskatoon University in Canada.) And so any thoughts that I might have had of becoming a chest physician had to be put aside on a permanent basis.

Nevertheless my postgraduate training had equipped me to embark on a career as a public health physician, especially as I saw it as an opportunity to remain within the broader field of the prevention and control of communicable diseases and so, after a brief spell in child health work in London, I became Deputy Medical Officer of Health of the Borough of Reigate in Surrey. Appropriately enough, my first epidemiological task there was to deal with an outbreak of tuberculosis in a primary school, which would involve tuberculin testing of the children and X-raying the staff. Before beginning this investigation I was given an extremely valuable piece of advice by my chief, Dr Tom Bingham (the father of England's future Lord Chief Justice Bingham), who said something along the following lines. "When you arrange to X-ray the staff, you'll probably find that one or two don't actually turn up on the day. Pursue them especially, and if you find that there's still one missing *pursue that person in particular*." As a result of my following this advice to the letter, a member of the teaching staff was found to have open tuberculosis. At first I was nonplussed as I knew that schoolteachers had to have a pre-employment chest X-ray but I was then informed that the individual was a temporary "supply" teacher and, incredibly, at that time such personnel were not required to be screened. Very soon thereafter I was being taught the practical aspects of giving BCG vaccine by intradermal injection, the most valuable method of offering *primary* protection against the disease. My teacher was Dr Tom Pollock (no relation, unfortunately for me!) the Head of the Medical Research Council's Tuberculosis Research Unit.

It would have been difficult to believe, then in the late 1950s, that tuberculosis would not be virtually eradicated as an endemic disease in England within a couple of decades. However, three factors would soon shatter any tendency to such complacency—a greatly increased rate of immigration from countries with a high incidence of tuberculosis, the emergence of multi-drug resistance, and the complicating factor of HIV infection. I have dealt with this new situation in the final chapter.

Chapter 5
Dawn and Sunset

By the end of the war, there was an expectation of better social conditions for all in the country. Community health needed to be a major part of this perspective. Chapter 3 clearly portrayed the pre-war Medical Officer of Health as the head of a local department whose long-standing central function had been the prevention and control of communicable diseases and other environmental hazards. Other responsibilities had come and gone and more changes in the role would follow. In the post-war situation, some far-seeing holders of the office were beginning to view preventive medicine in a wider context and "social medicine" and "social and preventive medicine" were terms which were found alongside "public health," the implication being that the behaviour of the individual within society had an important bearing on health. The term should really have been *societal* medicine—i.e. medicine of society (Richardson 1956), but that would have been too clumsy. It would, however, have prevented the confusion with *socialised* medicine!

From about 1943, after much political and professional discussion, occasionally acrimonious, the result was the creation of a cluster of social welfare legislation—the creation of the Welfare State—designed to eliminate deprivation, and to promote, maintain and protect individual, family and community health and well-being.

The health component of this legislative package took the form of the National Health Service Act 1946, an instrument which had come about as a result of a bringing together of traditional concerns for health care emanating from voluntary, religious and philanthropic activities which had been in evidence since the nineteenth century. The overall goal was to provide for the establishment of a comprehensive health service available to all and, generally speaking, free of charge at the point of delivery. Few would have believed that such a service could really be "free" but there was probably incomplete understanding on the part of the public of the actual funding arrangements, i.e. principally out of general taxation and to a lesser extent from National Insurance payments. Certainly anecdotal evidence at the time suggested that the latter was believed to be the main source—entitlement arising from payment of "the stamp."

G. Pollock, *An Epidemiological Odyssey: The Evolution of Communicable Disease Control*, DOI 10.1007/978-94-007-3998-7_5,

The Minister of Health was charged to promote the establishment of such a service "designed to secure the improvement in the physical and mental health of the people and the prevention, diagnosis and treatment of illness." The question of the service being "available to all" meant, among other things, that hospital resources had to be spread as evenly as possible throughout the country. To this end, 14 Regional Hospital Boards were set up to cover the whole of England and within each region Hospital Management Committees were set up to administer local hospitals on a day-to-day basis. While the national strategy was determined by Central Government, the service was to be regionally organised and locally administered.

The coming into being of the National Health Service in England represented a major enterprise about which a great deal has already been written over the years. Accordingly it is not proposed to write further about it, in this work, except in as much as it concerned the control of communicable diseases. For example, a major outcome of these fundamental organisational changes was the fact that the Medical Officer of Health was no longer responsible for the management of the municipal hospitals (mainly long-stay establishments for the elderly, the mentally handicapped, and the mentally ill) which were now transferred to the relevant Regional Hospital Board. Although many individuals so professionally affected no doubt felt a sense of loss, or even grievance, at this reassignment, the positive side of the equation was that the Medical Officer of Health now had much more clear-cut responsibility in the field of prevention and community health for a defined population. Certainly, with the support of a small medical staff, a large community nursing force, the expertise of a team of public health inspectors, and the back-up of the Public Health Laboratory Service, he was well placed to make a serious contribution to the surveillance, prevention and control of communicable diseases in his locality. Moreover this essentially epidemiological function was not one which could reasonably be provided by hospitals or general practitioners and therefore there was no professional opposition to the Medical Officer of Health having these responsibilities. (It is perhaps worth pointing this out as many general practitioners disapproved of the continuation of the community child and school health services under the local authority umbrella in an era in which each individual now had, at least theoretically, free access to both general practitioner and hospital services.)

Since the creation of the post in the nineteenth century, principally to control infectious diseases and other environmental hazards, various developments had resulted in many other responsibilities being added, but the opportunities for rationalisation which now arose in this post-war setting allowed many of these to be reassigned to other authorities considered more appropriate, while consolidating others under the "umbrella" of the Medical Officer of Health. It can be seen, therefore, that communicable disease control had emerged as a major, central, continuous theme and on-going raison d'être of the post. A moment's reflection shows that this tradition had, in fact, already lasted about two and a half thousand years, since the City States of Classical Greece appointed municipal physicians to advise on the health of the local community and to deal with epidemics.

The measures available to the Medical Officer of Health for disease control were, by this time, considerable and had been growing and developing over a very long period, taking advantage of scientific discoveries and involving the law when necessary, mostly in a permissive or authorising sense but very rarely for enforcement purposes. These measures related to the possibility of infection from patients, contacts or carriers, generally spread by respiratory or gastrointestinal routes, or by contagious skin conditions. Indirect transmission of infection was, of course, progressively being prevented and controlled by scientific and technical developments rather than by the personal involvement of the Medical Officer of Health as in, for example, purification of public water supplies, pasteurisation of milk and introduction of hygienic food practices.

This, then, represented the structure of the local authority public health service when I moved to Stockport, an industrial town in North Cheshire, in 1961, as Deputy to the Medical Officer of Health, Dr Alexander Moir. Although my stay in that town was less than 2 years, it was a valuable traineeship in that it allowed me to participate in two episodes of considerable public health importance—the experience of vaccinating smallpox contacts and keeping them under surveillance when the disease erupted in the nearby city of Bradford, and the introduction of oral vaccination against poliomyelitis.

Between December 1961 and April 1962 a severe epidemic of smallpox in Karachi was responsible for five separate importations of the disease into England and Wales. Although the situation in Pakistan was known to the authorities, and large numbers of immigrants from that country were arriving in the UK by charter flight and minimal fares, there was no increase in airport health control measures until after the first imported case had been reported. In all, 67 cases occurred with 26 deaths (BMJ Editorial 1963). The outbreak in Bradford came to light on 11th January 1962 after the death of a patient in St Luke's Hospital. By rapid epidemiological investigation a further nine cases were discovered within 72 h. Contacts received vaccination and were kept under surveillance. Although mass vaccination of the public was not generally recommended, a variety of circumstances justified catering for the public demand for this protection and, in fact, approximately 250,000 people received vaccination within a 5 day period (Douglas and Edgar 1962). Full details of the outbreak had been sent to the Medical Officers of Health of neighbouring authorities within 48 h of the onset of the outbreak, and the media publicity led to a similar demand for mass vaccination sessions in Stockport.

In all, nearly 13,000 persons in the latter town were vaccinated or revaccinated as a result of the anxiety created by the nearby outbreak (Moir 1962). Fortunately two-thirds of these were carried out by the patients' own general practitioner, thereby allowing consideration of any possible contraindication to the procedure. The remaining third were dealt with by Dr Moir and his medical staff at local health authority clinics, including a number of "walk-in" mass vaccination sessions in the main hall of the health department headquarters. Although the best precautions were taken to question those attending the latter concerning possible contraindications, it was difficult in the circumstances—large numbers of anxious people queuing to be vaccinated—to guarantee the standard of screening which one would have desired. In spite of this, I can recall only one case of a serious complication. A middle-aged man had omitted to mention that he was on cortisone treatment and in consequence the vaccination "ran wild," spreading locally to form a lesion about 4 in. in diameter. He was immediately admitted to hospital for intensive treatment and had to have a skin graft to his upper arm. In this respect Stockport was indeed fortunate as, of the millions of people who were vaccinated in response to the outbreaks of the disease in 1961/1962, nearly as many people died from complications of vaccination as from smallpox itself (Pennington 2002). This experience offered an opportunity for both national and local publicity to be given to the need for parents to secure routine vaccination of infants at the appropriate age. (One has to remember that, at this time, the global eradication of smallpox, and the consequent end of the need for vaccination, were not to occur for nearly two further decades.)

The fact that this fatal disease had been imported from Pakistan over a relatively short period led to a growing public awareness of the association between disease and Commonwealth immigration at a time when a political debate was raging over the proposed Commonwealth Immigrants Bill. Unemployment had been the main focus of concern but now the whole question of health checks for immigrants was dealt with vigorously by the Press (Butterworth 1966). Bivins (2007) expressed the view that media reporting—in Pakistan, in addition to Britain—"*immediately entwined legislation and outbreak*." Nevertheless it was not until 1965 that the Ministry of Health in London wrote to all Medical Officers of Health stressing the importance of all such immigrants being visited so that they could be given general information about the health services and persuaded to arrange to become registered with a general practitioner with a view particularly to having a chest X-ray carried out (Ministry of Health 1965a). A broadly similar letter was sent to all general practitioners themselves (Ministry of Health 1965b). It was clear that this was focused on detecting tuberculosis—admittedly becoming a significant problem—,the question of quarantinable diseases being left to the airport health authorities in accordance with the Public Health (Aircraft) Regulations.

Although vaccination against poliomyelitis had been available in England since 1956, the antigen, developed by Dr Jonas Salk, was an inactivated one which offered only approximately 80% protection against the disease. This vaccine had not, in fact, been free from problems initially. Just 15 days after the 1955 clinical trials in the United States had pronounced the vaccine "safe," a number of vaccinated children developed poliomyelitis. Staff of the Public Health Service's Communicable Disease Center were rapidly able to trace the outbreak to seven lots of vaccine manufactured by Cutter Laboratories in California which contained some live vaccine. As a result, 204 cases of poliomyelitis were traced to this quality control failure. Three quarters of these were paralytic and 11 died (McGrew 1985). The "Cutter Incident" led immediately to improved control measures by pharmaceutical manufacturers but, on reflection, and taking into account contemporary attitudes to vaccine safety, one might consider it surprising that the Salk vaccine was used so widely so soon after the tragedy. Perhaps the fear of the actual disease itself was the powerful incentive. It has to be recalled that, during the early 1950s, as many as around 8,000 cases were notified annually in the United Kingdom alone (Salisbury et al. 2006).

The new vaccine—a live one—developed by Dr Albert Sabin, was considered to offer a very much higher level of protection—around 99%. Dr Sabin visited London in February 1963 to try to interest Medical Officers of Health in his new vaccine. I was fortunate in that Dr Moir sent me to represent him at this meeting, showing what I considered to be a touching (but probably undeserved) faith in me by saying "If you're convinced by the evidence, go straight ahead and order enough of the vaccine to meet Stockport's requirements. It would be good to be the first local health authority to use it." I did exactly as he had requested but the episode had an interesting and, in retrospect, amusing sequel. When the packages arrived from the manufacturer and were place in the basement of the central health clinic for temporary storage, the building's cleaning staff refused to enter the area as they had heard (correctly) that this was a "live" vaccine and were nervous about possibly coming into contact with "something invisible crawling about the place" as one of them expressed it! Some intensive negotiations with their Trade Union representatives were necessary before this hurdle could be cleared. In addition to the higher level of protection, another benefit of using this vaccine, especially appreciated by children, was that the procedure did not require an injection, being administered as three drops on a sugar lump.

The following year 1964 brought a degree of notoriety to my home town of Aberdeen in that it became the focus of a major outbreak of typhoid fever, with a total of 476 cases. All were traced to the consumption of cooked meats purchased from a shop in the city centre. Detailed investigation revealed that the infection originated from a large tin of corned beef which had been opened in the shop and sold in slices. Failure to clean the meat-slicer adequately meant that some other cooked meats subsequently became contaminated and therefore were also capable of spreading the infection. The large tin of corned beef had been imported from a meat canning factory in South America where it was discovered that, after heat treatment, the cans had been cooled by being plunged into a tank filled with raw river water from which typhoid bacilli could be isolated. Bacilli had obviously been drawn into the can during cooling. This episode led to the United Kingdom enforcing local food hygiene standards for those food-processing factories overseas wishing to export to Britain (Milne 1964).

Only a few months before the Aberdeen outbreak, I had had to deal with my own (very limited) typhoid episode in the City of Coventry, to which I had moved in 1963 as Deputy to the Medical Officer of Health there, Dr T Morrison Clayton. The person affected had only recently returned from a holiday in Sardinia and the evidence suggested that she had been infected in that country. She was admitted to the local Whitley Isolation Hospital and eight persons who had had fairly close contact with her were placed under careful surveillance for a period of 3 weeks. Fortunately no subsequent cases occurred from this source. (However this episode *did* teach me a valuable lesson in epidemiological history-taking, namely that some people might not necessarily take kindly, for whatever reason, to being asked detailed questions about their recent movements, and one had to be sensitive to this!)

In the 1960s the disease known at that time as Infective Hepatitis (now known as Hepatitis A) was causing many problems and had been frequently referred to in England as "the most important unsolved problem in the field of infectious diseases." The fact that the disease was not notifiable in England meant that there was little in the way of epidemiological information which could aid understanding. Accordingly a number of local health authorities sought permission for the condition to be made locally notifiable, Coventry being one of these. It was felt that such an arrangement would help to prevent spread of infection from notified cases and would also shed some light on the natural history of the infection. An important feature of the latter, for example, was the difficulty in making a distinction between this disease and another condition known at the time as Serum Hepatitis (now known as Hepatitis B) which could be conveyed by human blood, either through contaminated syringes and needles or blood transfusion procedures (Clayton 1963). One small episode is perhaps worth reporting. A localised outbreak of Infective Hepatitis occurred in 1963 in the City Health Department's Junior Training Centre for children with severe learning difficulties. This had not responded to the usual methods of control and it was decided to try the effect of giving gamma-globulin to all the children at the Centre who had not experienced a clinical attack. It was gratifying that from that point no further cases occurred, but one had to admit that other factors, such as all the susceptibles already being exhausted, could also have played a part in this outcome. The publication of this novel approach (Pollock 1964) led to a certain amount of international interest and a senior public health physician from the Netherlands Institute for Preventive Medicine visited Coventry to discuss it in detail. This led indirectly to my subsequently being awarded a Council of Europe Travelling Fellowship to study the provision of public health services in the cities of Amsterdam and Utrecht, leading in turn to the development of strong professional links between Coventry City Health Department and the Ministry of Public Health and Social Affairs (*Ministerie van Volksgesondheid en Sociale Zaken*) in the Netherlands

The following year also put Coventry on the "epidemiological map" for a limited time. In January 1964 a dozen or so girls aged 12–14 years in three separate classrooms in a secondary modern school became suddenly ill with nausea, giddiness and collapse. There was no evidence of a toxic gas or inadequate ventilation and the symptoms were not related to the taking of school meals or school milk. Further cases occurred over the next few days and similar outbreaks involving both girls and boys began to affect two other schools in the city. Two of the schools were closed for a 2 week period, after which no further cases occurred, but the third school continued to be affected to a limited extent for a further 2 weeks. From start to finish the incident lasted 45 days and involved 404 pupils and two members of staff.

The affected pupils were quite ill, most having to be sent home by ambulance where the majority recovered after about 3 days, although in a quarter of instances similar illnesses occurred in both adults and pre-school children at home. Laboratory investigations were completely negative: no virus was grown from culture of throat swabs and no pathogens were found in samples of school meals, school milk or tuck-shop confectionery. The illness remained a mystery. In many ways the clinical picture resembled the group of conditions described variously in medical literature as "epidemic vertigo," "epidemic nausea" and "winter vomiting disease," but the term "epidemic collapse" was used for the first time as actual collapse was the most striking feature. When a paper on the incident appeared in the British Medical

Journal (Pollock and Clayton 1964) responses were evenly balanced between those who felt that it was an infection caused by an undetermined virus (norovirus was not identified until 1968), and those who were convinced that it should have been called "epidemic hysteria."

There was an interesting tailpiece to the event. Many years later I received a telephone call from the International Division of the Department of Health in London which had been contacted by a health administration in Israel. Apparently a number of Palestinian girls in a secondary school on the occupied Left Bank had suddenly demonstrated similar symptoms to those experienced in the Coventry outbreak and the Palestinian authorities had raised concerns that the school water supply might have been deliberately poisoned. Understandably the Israelis were anxious to show that such symptoms could readily occur from virus infection or hysteria and they were trying to collect as much information as possible from published work in this field. I gave as many details of the Coventry incident as I could recall but, perhaps not surprisingly, I was never informed of the outcome of this delicate situation.

Two further Coventry incidents from the 1960s are worthy of brief mention, firstly because they occurred at a time when it could have been expected that immunisation would have prevented such infections, but more importantly because they happened shortly before legislation was due to dismantle the established structure for communicable disease control in England.

In June 1967 a case of paralytic poliomyelitis was notified from the Whitley Isolation Hospital. The patient was a two and a half-year old girl with paralysis in both arms. In accordance with the official guidance at that time, not only the family members but also all the children in the neighbourhood, and those attending the same day nursery as the patient, were immediately given a single dose of oral poliovaccine. I recall the event very clearly as the day took on a certain festive atmosphere. The weather was sunny and very warm and mothers stood with their babies and young children at the doors of their terraced houses awaiting the "sugar lump with the pink drops." Cooperation was 100%. The puzzling feature of the case was that the patient had previously received a full course of oral poliovaccine and thus should have been completely immune to poliomyelitis. What the Coventry Public Health Laboratory actually grew were Herpes Simplex virus from her throat swab and Coxsackie A16 virus from her faeces. The view of the PHLS was that this was a case of "paralytic poliomyelitis" caused by the Coxsackie A16 virus. The local publicity concerning the episode had to be handled carefully, otherwise the community could have been left with the impression that the polio vaccination programme was of no value.

In July of the following year an 11 year old boy was diagnosed as a case of diphtheria when a swab from his sore throat grew a toxigenic strain of *C. Diphtheriae.* The surprising feature of this case was that he had *not* been immunised, even although free immunisation facilities were readily at hand. [The reasons why some children needlessly miss out on routine immunisation are discussed later in this work.] The patient was quite ill and developed paralysis of the soft palate as a complication. Investigation showed that his parents and two brothers were also harbouring the organism in the throat but were not ill. His siblings *had* been immunised and it was felt that both parents had pre-existing immunity from natural infection in childhood. All were treated in hospital until they were non-infectious. The most scrupulous investigation of contacts failed to reveal any carrier and there were no further cases. An aunt had recently visited on holiday from Cape Town and an attempt was made to ascertain from the Medical Officer of Health of that city whether this could have been the source of infection, but this did not prove to be a fruitful line of enquiry. The publicity arising from this case did, however, provide an excellent opportunity to remind the local community that diphtheria was a serious and potentially fatal disease and one which could be kept at bay only by routine active immunisation of children in infancy.

A further mention of Coventry in the 1960s relates to its, somewhat unexpectedly, having to take on the responsibilities of an airport health authority. Coventry Airport, at Baginton on the city's south-east border, had been an important RAF station during the Second World War but subsequently had become little more than a venue for private light aircraft, apart from the British United Airways services to Calais and occasional day-trips to the bulb fields in Holland. This changed dramatically in 1966 when *Air Charter Enterprises* began to use the airport as a base for their world-wide operations. It was their proud boast that, using their three large Lockheed Constellation aircraft, they would fly *anyone* or *anything* to *any* part of the world at *any* time of the day or night! As an example, they would carry freight to the Far East but bring back some British troops on leave or other persons prepared to have a less than comfortable but cheap flight, on the return journey. This meant that if the aircraft was returning from, for example, a country where smallpox was endemic, all crew and passengers had to be able to show valid vaccination certificates or else had to be vaccinated at the airport and placed under surveillance for 14 days in the area of the country to which they were proceeding. Hurriedly a miniscule health control unit was created in the terminal building comprising a small examination room equipped with a vaccine refrigerator, and a tiny isolation room (little more than a cupboard) in which any persons showing suspicious symptoms would be detained until the specially designated smallpox ambulance arrived to take them to an appropriate isolation hospital. The most memorable episode in connection with this unlikely set-up was in 1967 when a small group of Coventry industrialists returning from a business trip to Germany had to be placed under surveillance as a result of their having been in the locality of a small outbreak of so-called "Green Monkey Disease" (subsequently identified as Marburg virus disease).

Lastly in this sequence of Coventry in the field of prevention of communicable disease it is worth mentioning the establishment of its Yellow Fever Vaccination Clinic. By the mid-1960s many of the city's residents were already travelling further afield on holiday, on business trips, or to visit family members or friends in any part of the world. Vaccination against yellow fever is a formal requirement under the International Health Regulations for those travelling to, or through, the countries in the yellow fever endemic zone, essentially those in the tropical belt of Africa and South America. These Regulations laid down stringent requirements concerning the actual vaccination procedure… temperature control, time elapsed between mixing the vaccine and giving the injection etc., and yellow fever vaccination centres had to be authorised by WHO after satisfying the criteria demanded.

However the nearest centre for Coventry residents was in Birmingham City Health Department and data obtained from our Birmingham colleagues showed that the numbers attending there from Coventry and its immediate surroundings were quite substantial. Accordingly, a strong case was put to the Ministry of Health to ask WHO for permission to establish a centre in Coventry, assurances having been given that all the criteria re standards etc. would be met. The outcome was that the Coventry centre was able to open on 7th February 1968, initially operated by myself and offering a weekly service within the Occupational Health Unit in the New Council Offices. However as the demand for the service continued to grow—young persons trekking overland in the Developing World had joined the business and holiday travellers in needing this protection—I took the decision to move the centre to the outpatient department of the Coventry and Warwickshire Hospital in the city centre, a fact reported in the *Coventry Evening Telegraph* under the heading "The Coventry Yellow Peril Fighters Are Moving House!" From the outset the centre had rapidly developed into a general travel advisory service, offering much more than simply yellow fever vaccination, particularly drawing attention to the dangers of the different varieties of malaria and the means of preventing them.

[The strict criteria demanded by WHO for the establishment of such a centre were also reflected within the Armed Services in that one had to be of consultant-equivalent status to operate such a service, e.g. a Lieutenant-Colonel in the Royal Army Medical Corps or a Wing Commander in the RAF Medical Branch. This led to one rather entertaining experience for me. In May 1955, as Regimental Medical Officer of the 1st Battalion, the King's Shropshire Light Infantry, I had arranged for the troops to receive their yellow fever vaccination at Whittington Barracks, Lichfield, prior to our embarkation for Kenya because of the Mau Mau uprising there. (We were to be there "in aid of the civil power"—the political reason given.) The Assistant Director of Army Pathology for the Midlands, a charming Maltese Lieutenant-Colonel whom I knew well, was due to take an entire day to carry out the task but the evening before he was due to arrive he telephoned me from Chester, sounding hoarse and very ill, to say that he was incapacitated by influenza and unable to leave his bed. The event could not be postponed; the unit was under embarkation orders and the vaccine was due to be delivered in its specialised vehicle. The only possibility at such short notice was that I should carry out the procedures personally, a simple enough task but my rank was only that of Captain. In order to satisfy the International Health Regulations it was agreed, after many telephone calls, that I would assume the (acting) rank of Lieutenant-Colonel for 1 day. The troops were highly delighted at my promotion but unfortunately the brief elevation was not reflected in my pay cheque!]

Moving back from these purely local events to consideration of more general issues, it is reasonable to ask at this point: what brought to an end the clear-cut responsibility for the prevention and control of communicable disease in England? The first hint of the major changes came in the Government's 1968 "Green Paper" (at that time a relatively unfamiliar term for a consultative document) entitled

The Administrative Structure of the Medical and Related Services in England and Wales. (Ministry of Health 1968). In the Foreword the Minister of Health, Kenneth Robinson, gave it as his view that the organisation of health services had progressed almost as far as possible within the existing divided administrative structure and that the time had come for that structure as a whole to be radically reconsidered. The paramount requirement, in his view, was that all the different kinds of care and treatment that an individual might need should be readily available and that this would require the closest collaboration not only between doctors, nurses and other workers, but also between those who provided and those who administered the various services. His suggested solution, which he made the central theme of the document, was the unified administration of the medical and related services in an area by one authority, in place of the multiplicity of authorities concerned in the existing arrangements.

Understandably, the main thrust of the proposals concerned the integration of local hospital and community health services which meant, in effect, setting up a new area authority which would have comprehensive scope for coordinating the policy and operation of a wide range of services. Within this broad concept, the community health services were largely identified as domiciliary midwifery, child health clinics, home nursing, health visiting and immunisation—essentially personal health services which, it was felt, might benefit from being provided alongside, or in closer association with, the family doctor service.

Against this background, the future role of the Medical Officer of Health was seen as that of a "community physician" whose duties might be extended to include the epidemiological evaluation of the standards of health in each area, *but who would still need to be responsible for the prevention and control of communicable disease* (my italics). In fact, the 1968 Green Paper emphasised that this latter responsibility should be clear and that there should be continuous and effective surveillance of communicable disease in the community, with prompt and skilful investigation of suspicious circumstances and firm measures to prevent, limit and control the spread of disease. If the area authority were felt to be the appropriate means of deploying in a single organisation all the medical and related skills involved in public health activity, then the community physicians concerned were considered well placed to work in close collaboration with family doctors, hospitals and the Public Health Laboratory Service. Attention was drawn, however, to the need to define in due course the precise dividing line between the public health function of a new area authority and the related functions of the local authority, which would have to await decisions on the future organisation of local government.

The second Green Paper, *The Future Structure of the National Health Service* (Department of Health and Social Security 1970), introduced by the Secretary of State, Richard Crossman, was able to take into account not only the comments received from the original consultative process but the also the contents of the White Paper (the Government's stated intentions) on local government reorganisation. The concept of an area health authority appeared to have been consolidated, with a careful delineation of the administrative boundary which would have to be drawn between the National Health Service and the public health and social service functions of the local authority. In fact, there seemed to be much more concern about the latter of these two local authority services, especially the potential overlap of health provision and social care, and less about the prevention and control of communicable diseases which, the document stated, although previously "the major cause of death of people of working age ***have now been virtually eliminated as health problems***" (my italics).

Local authorities were to retain their responsibilities for the prevention of spread of communicable diseases, food safety and hygiene, and port health, with medical staff of the area health authority collaborating with the local authority's environmental health officers, especially for the control of outbreaks of communicable disease or food poisoning. The Medical Officer of Health was to become the chief "community physician" and provide medical and epidemiological advice to both the area health authority and the local authority although, for the first time since 1888, a postgraduate qualification in this specialised field of work would no longer be a statutory requirement. It was beginning to appear that the separation of the successor to the Medical Officer of Health from the "need to be responsible for the prevention and control of communicable disease—and the prompt and skilful investigation of suspicious circumstances and firm measures to prevent, limit and control.........etc." was implicit in the proposed reorganisation. Much had changed during a period of 2 years, and many in the field felt that this probably reflected the considered views on priorities of those providing medical advice to the Secretary of State.

A third publication, *National Health Service Reorganisation: Consultative Document* (Department of Health and Social Security 1971), focused almost exclusively on the proposed management arrangements. (It has to be recalled that management theory and new definitions of "effectiveness" and "efficiency" had dominated discussions on public sector management throughout the 1960s, along with a variety of so-called management techniques imported from the United States, initially into British industry and commerce and subsequently into the public sector. Now the word "management" had become a mystique) **Communicable disease prevention and control were not mentioned at all**, although reference was made to the necessity to ensure that local authorities continued to have the medical advice they needed "for the effective discharge of their functions in...............the environmental health services." This advice was to be provided by a health authority doctor who was to be known as the Medical Officer for Environmental Health (MOEH). A fourth Green Paper, a White Paper and a Bill followed in rapid succession with no specific reference to communicable disease control and so this key issue was missing when the National Health Service Reorganisation Act itself appeared in 1973. The post of Medical Officer of Health itself was to cease to exist as from 1 April 1974, when the reorganised National Health Service came into being. **Thus the arrangements which had been carefully built up for over a century were to be dismantled—a casualty of a reorganisation clearly focused elsewhere.**

Some guidance from the Government during 1973 and early 1974 attempted to explain how the reorganised services would operate. One of these communications (Department of Health and Social Security 1973), specifically covering the control of notifiable diseases and food poisoning, appeared to acknowledge the possibility of urgent problems arising in this field as it referred to the need for relevant staff to be ready to carry out their responsibilities "on a 24-h basis as from midnight 31 March 1974." One key event necessitating the issue of this emergency guidance was a limited outbreak of smallpox in London in March and April 1973. A laboratory technician working part-time in the pox virus laboratory at the London School of Hygiene and Tropical Medicine became ill on 11 March and saw her own family doctor 2 days later, having reported the matter to the two microbiologists to whom she was accountable. No one at the time associated her illness with her work and she was admitted to a general ward at St Mary's Hospital, Harrow road, with a diagnosis of pyrexia of unknown origin. This led in due course to the deaths from smallpox of two persons who visited that ward. The Committee of Inquiry Report on this incident (Department of Health and Social Security 1974) made the point that no one had grasped the true nature of the emergency because of lack of experience in smallpox and its control. The considerable publicity given to this outbreak by the media at the time had the effect of lowering the threshold for public alarm in relation to the disease. Having not heard anything about smallpox for over a decade, the public was suddenly and uncomfortably reminded of its existence, at the same time as being aware of continuing immigration from countries in which the condition was still endemic, especially the Indian Sub-Continent. It was against this background that a national alert was sparked off by the notification of a case in Coventry, leading to my personal involvement as Medical Officer of Health, as is described in detail below.

On 21st April 1973, the Saturday of a Bank Holiday weekend, I was telephoned by a general practitioner to notify what he considered to be a case of smallpox, a 20 month old boy. The doctor was Asian and informed me that he was very familiar with the clinical appearance of the disease, having seen many cases in his own country. I immediately visited the child's home and agreed that the clinical features suggested smallpox and that, taking account of the family's recent movements, appropriate action should be taken forthwith. The boy, born in Coventry of Indian parents, had returned to the city in the early hours of that day after spending a holiday in India with his mother. They had been met at Heathrow Airport by the father who drove them home via the M1 motorway, stopping at the Newport Pagnell service area where they had a meal in the self-service restaurant. Before formal action could be taken to admit a patient to a designated smallpox hospital, one of the Department of Health's smallpox consultants was required to examine the patient in order to confirm the diagnosis and so I telephoned the duty consultant, a charming and distinguished professor, at his home in Birmingham. On examination he also regarded the case as confirmed on clinical grounds and advised me to ask the Regional Health Authority to mobilise its small specialised smallpox unit at St Catherine-de-Barnes, near Birmingham, immediately. (The term "mobilise" requires a brief word of explanation. The hospital was not in regular use but could be brought into operation, with its entire staff, literally within hours.) The boy was admitted to that hospital on the same evening.

Having secured the isolation of the actual case I then had to turn my urgent attention to the boy's contacts who, as far as could be determined, consisted only of his immediate family—four adults and five children. Although all had valid vaccination certificates, as they frequently travelled to India, I revaccinated the entire family, just to be absolutely sure. This was not an occasion for having any doubts! I carefully explained to them that they must remain in quarantine in the family home for the incubation period of the disease and that they could receive no visitors. I felt it necessary to stress this point as it would have been totally understandable for family and friends to visit them following their return from India and I had no intention of allowing infection to spread within the city or further afield.

To emphasise the importance of preventing such spread I took the rather unusual step, *with the family's informed consent*, of locking both the front and back doors of the house and arranging for food etc. supplies to be delivered through the ground-floor front window by members of my own staff, all of whom had been regularly revaccinated. The media made much of this unprecedented situation and pictures of the street appeared on regional television with references to the "beleaguered home!" However the message which the media were conveying was unhesitatingly one of total support, with frequent references to the obvious care which was being taken to protect the local population. It has to be recalled that there had been the smallpox incident in London as recently as earlier that month. In spite of their support, however, dealing with the media took up an inordinate amount of my time especially as the Department of Health had put out a national alert on the grounds that persons visiting the Newport Pagnell service area at the relevant time could have been exposed to infection. Apart from dealing with enquiries from the Press I had to appear on regional and national television at a time when I would have preferred to be devoting all my energies to keeping the contacts under twice daily surveillance. The compromise which I reached in due course was to leave a written statement with the young woman who, with her small team, provided me with all the administrative support which I required while I did the actual fieldwork. (It says a great deal for their commitment that, when contacted by telephone, all had promptly agreed to give up their Bank Holiday weekend and report immediately for duty.)

In the event, on the evening of Wednesday 25th April, the final results of laboratory investigations showed that the boy was *not*, in fact, suffering from smallpox, but rather from an unusual form of measles along with a quite separate skin condition which, in combination, closely resembled the clinical picture of smallpox. It is interesting to note that the Press response to this news reflected only the sheer relief that the local population had not been exposed to risk. There were no criticisms of "over-reaction" or unjustified actions. The *Coventry Evening Telegraph* front page headline read "ALL CLEAR ON SMALLPOX SUSPECT" and its Editorial commented on the reassurance that Coventry citizens must feel that, even over a Bank Holiday weekend, a vigilant City Health Department was ready and able to take prompt action to protect their health. The relevant staff modestly accepted this tribute.

The question of legal authority in cases of this kind needs to be considered in a little detail. Although it was with the family's informed consent that I locked the doors of their home and, not only was I not criticised by anyone for taking this unusual step, I was actually generally commended for my thoroughness. I was quietly horrified to be told, quite informally by a legal friend years afterwards, that I could have been guilty of a number of offences ranging from illegal detention to ignoring fire risk. But circumstances alter cases. At the time, the law on the control of infectious diseases was very outdated, with parts going back to the previous century. It allowed the Medical Officer of Health, *inter alia*, to require the admission of an infectious individual to hospital and, if necessary, detention there. But (almost certainly because of an oversight) there was no legal authority to enforce surveillance of contacts, or isolation of cases or quarantine of contacts at home—absolutely central activities of communicable disease control (Button J, 1999, Public health legal information unit, Matlock, Derbyshire. Personal communication. Telephone conversation 11th January 1999). It is certainly fortunate that the great majority of persons are readily cooperative with regard to public health activities designed to prevent the spread of infection, provided that these measures are explained adequately to them. An interesting thought—perhaps everyone involved in such a situation assumes that such legal authority *does* exist and behaves accordingly?

What needs to be realised, however, is that, in cities like Coventry with a significant proportion of persons from the Indian Sub-Continent, such events were quite common and, had there not been the need for a national alert because of the Newport Pagnell involvement, the media might never have known about the episode. The sequence of events was commonly as follows. A general practitioner would be concerned at being called to see a patient recently arrived from the Sub-Continent with a combination of fever and a rash suggestive of early smallpox, i.e. especially on the face, hands, wrists, feet and ankles. On being notified of this, I would visit the patient, take specimens from the rash and immediately have them examined at the virus laboratory in Birmingham which, at that time, was the only one equipped with an electron microscope and where I had an excellent working relationship with the professor of virology. Fortunately the findings were invariably reassuring but I wondered why this clinical presentation was so common and it was only when I had begun to take careful *travel* histories, and had acquired a knowledge of *very* basic Urdu/Punjabi by attending a course at a local college, that I understood the explanation given by a number of returning travellers. The usual story was that people returning to Coventry from a family holiday in, for example, Punjab would travel overnight to Delhi Airport in an open bus, wearing light clothing but with face, hands and ankles exposed to flies and other biting insects. This meant that on arrival in this country there could be some insect bite marks with a similar distribution to a smallpox eruption. It only needed the individual to have a degree of fever from e.g. an upper respiratory infection for the clinical picture to be very suggestive, and therefore the source of a certain amount of alarm.

Chapter 6
A Need for Damage Limitation

The new integrated hospital and community health services were, as mentioned in the previous chapter, to be provided by an "Area Health Authority," the territory covered to be coterminous with that of the matching local authority. This approach had only a limited existence, as it was found to be unwieldy (some said unworkable), and it was therefore replaced in due course by the concept of a District Health Authority (DHA), covering a population of around 200,000–300,000 and forming a natural unit of a District General Hospital (DGH) along with its catchment population, served by linked community health services. In the run-up to NHS reorganisation, the Government and relevant representatives of the medical profession had agreed a new staffing structure for doctors who had, up to that point, held senior positions in the public health service or in hospital administration, following the recommendations of the Hunter Report (Department of Health and Social Security 1972). From April 1974 these doctors were to members of a new specialty to be known as "community medicine"—the rationale being that these "community physicians" (the career grade to be that of "specialist in community medicine," one of whom would be the Medical Officer for Environmental Health—the MOEH) would bring their diagnostic professional skills to determining the health problems of populations rather than those of individual patients. "Treatment" and "prevention," for example, would be represented by the organised actions taken to tackle these problems, or the provision of community services of a preventive or screening nature such as childhood immunisation and cervical cytology.

Much of this was, of course, not new, having been previously provided by the Medical Officer of Health's department. What *was* new was the fact that the ex-Medical Officer of Health was now also to be part of a consensus-forming Management Team with joint responsibility for managing the integrated hospital and community services at local level. Not all ex-Medical Officers of Health felt totally comfortable about working in a consensus team instead of being a Head of Department. In my new role as District Medical Officer for Coventry, for example, I personally had many reservations about the arrangement and it was therefore somewhat ironical that, because of my modest ability in spoken French, I was

G. Pollock, *An Epidemiological Odyssey: The Evolution of Communicable Disease Control*, DOI 10.1007/978-94-007-3998-7_6,

invited to speak in praise of this new set-up at international conferences at the francophone Université de Montréal (Pollock 1984), and in Lyon (Pollock 1988). Organisational relationships within the specialty of community medicine (later to be called public health medicine) were rather vague and imprecise. As the specialists were all of consultant-equivalent status, there could be no question of managerial accountability, and the ex-Medical Officer of Health, now Area Medical Officer and subsequently District Medical Officer (DMO), was required to "monitor and coordinate" their work (for which additional responsibility a salary supplement was payable). Agreed definitions for these terms were hard to come by, although it was often quietly and mischievously observed that "coordination was the term one used when one wished to conceal the nature of the activity being carried out!"

It would have been too much to hope for that these new arrangements for communicable disease control, hastily brought into being as part of a major management-focused reorganisation of the National Health Service, would operate smoothly and effectively, and indeed they did not. Among the difficulties with which the new MOsEH had to contend were: lack of staff support, the uncomfortable feeling that they were uneasily positioned between the National Health Service and the local authority environmental health department, along with a general feeling of professional isolation. Even their organisational relationship with the DMO was somewhat vague. Their disquiet was well founded. The Medical Officer of Health had been the head of a large department well-staffed with public health doctors, health visitors, district nurses and environmental health officers; the MOEH was "out there" virtually on his own, dependent for support on the goodwill of staff who were now accountable to other heads of departments, e.g. the Chief Environmental Health Officer or the Chief Nursing Officer.

Furthermore, Richard Crossman's conclusion that communicable diseases had been virtually eliminated soon proved to have been a major miscalculation, as the country was very soon beginning to be alarmed by what were being referred to as "emerging and re-emerging infections." Apart from the London smallpox episode, a number of new (i.e. emerging) infections were beginning to be identified: *Rotavirus* infections in young children (1973), *Cryptosporidium* infections affecting public water supplies (1976), Lassa haemorrhagic fever emanating from West Africa but soon with imported cases in England (1976), *Campylobacter* food poisoning (1977), Ebola-Marburg haemorrhagic fever originating in central Africa but similarly soon brought into England (1977), Legionnaire's Disease, first identified in the United States in 1976 but soon also recognised in England, HIV/AIDS (1983), and Hepatitis C in needle-sharing drug misusers (1989) all "emerging" post-1974. During the same period, notifications of *Salmonella* food-poisoning, especially *S. Enteritidis*, and meningococcal infections greatly increased. Other infections significantly "*re*-emerging" during this period included Hepatitis B as a result of increasing injecting drug misuse, and tuberculosis deriving both from immigrants from high-prevalence countries and those with immune systems weakened as a result of HIV infection.

The combination of the alarm caused by these events (especially the smallpox and Lassa fever episodes) and the loss of expertise in handling such situations, brought about by the early retirement of experienced Medical Officers of Health, along with the massive increase in both scheduled and charter air travel, led to an acknowledgement of the need for a national epidemiological centre, a case which had been well argued even before the first of the Green Papers (Galbraith 1967). Accordingly in 1977 the PHLS set up, on behalf of the Department of Health and Social Security (DHSS), the Communicable Disease Surveillance Centre (CDSC) with Dr N.S. Galbraith as its first Director, essentially to carry out communicable disease surveillance nationally, to provide advice and assistance in the investigation and control of communicable disease, and latterly to assist in teaching and training in this field. On Galbraith's advice, the Centre was administered within the PHLS, rather than the DHSS, to promote the necessary collaboration between his staff and the adjoining microbiologists whose support would be of crucial importance.

The Centre began in a very modest way, consisting of a portacabin behind the PHLS headquarters. Apart from the Director there were no other epidemiologists on the staff, although for a limited period a senior medical officer from the DHSS was seconded to the unit—"to keep an eye on him" was Galbraith's genially tolerant view (Galbraith, 1982, Personal communication).This was perhaps in keeping with the general lack of encouragement from the DHSS and the PHLS itself, both of which had reservations about the value and indeed wisdom of this project. However it attracted the attention of Dr Alexander Langmuir, Head of the Epidemiology Department at CDC Atlanta, who, after visiting it, invited Dr Galbraith to visit his establishment. It was following this trip to the United States that Dr Galbraith introduced the teaching and training element in CDSC's responsibilities, as this function had not been envisaged by the DHSS when it agreed to the setting up of the Centre. In 1978, the year after its coming into being, CDSC was moved to improved accommodation on the PHLS site but it was only later that year, as a result of a smallpox outbreak in Birmingham, that the DHSS fully accepted the key importance of CDSC by virtue of the way in which the Centre had successfully dealt with the contacts in this episode (Galbraith 1998).

This Birmingham outbreak had represented an unforeseen tragedy. On Friday 11th August 1978 a medical photographer in the Anatomy Department at Birmingham University, which was located directly above the laboratory dealing with poxviruses, developed a headache and aching muscles. Three days later she developed a rash for which her general practitioner prescribed an antibiotic on the following day. She went to stay with her parents but, as her condition worsened, on 24th August she was admitted to hospital where smallpox was suspected, in spite of the fact that she had been vaccinated against this disease in 1966. This diagnosis was confirmed by electron microscopy. Although she was transferred immediately to the special smallpox hospital at St Catherine de Barnes she died on 11th September. Her mother also developed the disease but, having been vaccinated on 24th August, she recovered. It was concluded that the virus had travelled in air currents up a service duct. The Director of the laboratory, who was the University's Professor of Microbiology, was so distressed by this episode that he took his own life (Pennington 2002). Because of the time which had elapsed between the patient becoming infectious and subsequently being isolated, a large number of contacts had to be identified, sought out, vaccinated and then placed under surveillance. It was evident from CDSC's prompt and skilled actions that a new and reliable system of national surveillance had been put in place.

During his first few years as Director Dr Galbraith travelled to each Region in England to explain the role of the Centre and to promote good relationships with the key personnel at local level… public health doctors (especially MOsEH), microbiologists and clinicians This was particularly important from the point of view of reassuring MOsEH who, already uncertain enough about their position in the overall structure, were anxious not to be "over- lorded" by any national epidemiological service. His CDSC "road shows" mounted in each Region became well known, and were greatly looked forward to as they offered an exciting vision of potential developments in this field at a time when some staff might be becoming a little disenchanted by their career choice. His personal commitment to these appearances was all the more remarkable given that he had suffered from severe rheumatoid arthritis for most of his adult life and required crutches and a specially adapted car to get around. These events were also significant in that they encouraged many young public health doctors to become trainee epidemiologists, some by secondment to CDSC itself.

He was also keen to establish professional links with colleagues in other countries. Apart from the well-established connection with CDC Atlanta, he felt that it would also be of value to arrange some kind of exchange of ideas and even personnel with France, which in 1983 caused me to be personally involved, again because of my modest competence in the language of that country. Accordingly I was given the honorary title of "associate consultant epidemiologist" (which he felt "*would not upset anyone*!") and authorised to travel to Paris on CDSC's behalf to meet Professor Robert Netter, Director of the *Laboratoire National de la Santé*, to explore these possibilities. This visit had an interesting consequence for me personally as Professor Netter introduced me to a number of senior medical epidemiologists at the Ministry of Health in Paris, as a result of which I learned a great deal about the organisation of communicable disease control services in France. The main difference from English practice that I observed, at that time, was the strong degree of Central direction exercised by the medical epidemiologists in the Bureau of Infectious Diseases (*Bureau des Maladies Transmissibles*) within the Ministry over all local public health physicians concerning the control of outbreaks—what would perhaps nowadays be referred to as micro-management from Central Government. This would have been culturally unacceptable in England. As mentioned in Chap. 4, as far back as the establishment of the EPHLS in 1939, any advice or assistance from that organisation in relation to a local outbreak could only be offered at the request of, or with the consent of, the relevant Medical Officer of Health in whom the final responsibility was vested.

Brief reference has been made above to the unforeseen "cascade" of emerging and re-emerging infections which, by a sort of bitter irony, appeared to flow in the wake of the dismantling of the Medical Officer of Health's department in 1974. However the arrival of HIV/AIDS deserves a little more detailed attention. The gradual realisation in 1981 that certain immunodeficiency diseases, especially

Pneumocystis pneumonia, affecting homosexual men in California were due to a retrovirus (not actually identified until 1983) in no way heralded the global epidemic of HIV infection which was to come. Brandt (1987) expressed the view that the epidemic had begun at a moment of relative complacency and therefore that there was little social or political experience in confronting a public health crisis of this dimension.

In England the impact of understanding the nature of the infection was such that the Chief Medical Officer of the Department of Health in London, Sir Donald Acheson, called a meeting of all DMOs in April 1986 at which he informed them that this slow-burning epidemic would transform the day-to-day content of their professional lives and instructed them to return to their Districts and forthwith set up local coordinating committees to deploy what resources they could muster in the fight against this new disease. This timing turned out to be important as locally, as in most of the country by the late summer of that year, lack of clear information was leading to public concern about the possible means of spread of the infection. Public alarm and misinformation were equally rife. People were anxious about the possibility of being infected by such harmless activities as standing next to someone in a bus queue.

Accordingly, that autumn, in conjunction with the local media (mainly the *Coventry Evening Telegraph* and *Mercia Sound*), Coventry Health Authority, launched a major campaign of public information dissemination, spearheaded by myself as DMO, to explain in clear and unambiguous terms the nature of the infection, how it was spread, how it could *not* be spread, and how individuals could choose to behave in a way which carried a high risk or no risk at all. This clearly had to involve plain speaking on matters of sexual behaviour in a way which would probably have been unthinkable before that time. The core of the message was that HIV infection was a sexually transmitted disease which could also be spread by drug misusers who shared syringes or needles. Initially the media campaign was not totally straightforward. The Editor of the *Telegraph* was quite unhappy about using such explicit language, reminding me pointedly that this was a "family newspaper." (This situation was therefore very similar to that in 1942 when, as described in Chap. 4, the Wartime Government had to find ways of breaking the "taboo" on public discussion of sexual matters in its attempt to prevent and control VD.) However, as soon as Sir Donald Acheson had used the word "condom" during a televised debate on AIDS, it became respectable overnight and DMOs were able to use it, and indeed encouraged to do so in their various dealings with the media. Additionally, I asked a local consultant in genitourinary medicine to join with me and my medical and health education staff in addressing a large variety of local employers and other organisations, which in turn were able to pass on the facts to their employees or members. School medical officers and health visitors jointly worked with teaching staff to devise appropriate information-giving to pupils. Attention was drawn to the arrangements by which the Coventry Public Health Laboratory was offering a HIV screening service for persons who felt that they might have run the risk of being infected, and it was explained that such individuals would be offered both pre-test and post-test counselling as integral parts of the process. The former allowed the individual to think through the pros and cons of being tested and the latter gave an opportunity to review and discuss the individual's lifestyle in the case of a positive result.

As mentioned in Chap. 2, in an address to the Spring Conference of the Faculty of Community Medicine, Professor Michael Adler stated (1987): "Nowadays when one asks students: What disease has the following features: appeared suddenly, of American origin, sexual and vertical transmission, a carrier state, 2,000 deaths per year, and referred to as intended as a punishment for our sins and therefore a matter with which one should not interfere, they all answer AIDS. This is rather salutary since, as you will have realised, the disease is syphilis." Initially AIDS was portrayed by some of the media and consequently accepted by many of the public as something primarily affecting homosexual men—hence expressions such as "gay plague," as part of a general tendency to use members of this community as scapegoats. A senior police officer at that time was quoted on radio as referring to homosexuals as "swirling around in a cesspool of their own making." Therefore it was necessary to emphasise that infection by the transmission of blood and body fluids had equal relevance to both homosexual *and* heterosexual activity.

Concern was raised by some MOsEH on the question of DMOs, rather than themselves, being identified for this key coordinating role in what, after all, was clearly a matter of the control of a communicable disease. The official view, as far as this could be gleaned, seemed to be that the DMO, being part of the central management of the health authority, was likely to have a wider range of contacts with hospital consultants and health promotion staff etc., and to have greater access to the additional resources which might need to be mobilised. Again the question of professional hierarchy was being raised. Locally each situation had to be handled with sensitivity.

Writing now in 2011, it is difficult to recall how much misinformation there was about AIDS in the middle 1980s. A great many telephone calls were received from anxious individuals in Coventry who felt that they might have been placed at risk; the great majority, of course, had not even remotely been in any situation of risk. One such call came from the person in charge of a local Benefits Office. A disgruntled young man, on being refused some payment to which he felt entitled, spat on the desk and said: "I've got AIDS and now you'll all get it!" Another came from someone who said: "I know what a homosexual is, but what is a heterosexual?" The enquiry was a serious, not flippant, one and the answer could *not* be "Well, just *normal*." One had to make it clear that the word simply referred to sex between men and women, such was the need at that time for society to adjust to, and accept, the idea of differing sexual preference,

The setting up of CDSC had represented a major contribution to meeting many of the challenges of the time but a more fundamental response was soon to be brought about. This response represented a kind of paradox in that it was largely concerned with the organisation of communicable disease control *in the community* whereas the urgent need for it was triggered off by two *hospital* infection control failures.

At 7.00 am on Sunday 26th August 1984 a patient in Stanley Royd Hospital, Wakefield, a unit for the mentally ill and elderly mentally infirm, developed vomiting and diarrhoea. Within half an hour seven more patients in three separate wards had also presented with these symptoms. It very rapidly became obvious that a widespread outbreak of food poisoning was occurring as, shortly after the day nursing staff had arrived on the wards, there was a total on 36 cases on eight wards. It was unfortunate that the outbreak had begun on a Bank Holiday weekend with a number of key staff on holiday or away, including the Chairman of the hospital Cross Infection Committee and the MOEH (although the latter's deputy, the DMO, was able to be contacted.) By the time that the outbreak was over there had been a total of 461 cases with 19 deaths. It was concluded from the evidence that the outbreak had been caused by *Salmonella Typhimurium* infecting the meals served to the patients on the evening of Saturday 25th August 1984. A Public Inquiry set up to investigate this episode was critical not only of the hospital catering arrangements—"the preparation of food in an old, unworthy and unhealthy kitchen"—but also of medical and nursing management, especially because of their failure to seek help from outside specialists (Department of Health and Social Security 1986a). The result was that the Secretary of State for Social Services, Norman Fowler, decided to set up a Committee of Inquiry in to the Future Development of the Public Health Function and the Specialty of Community Medicine, to be chaired by the Government's Chief Medical Officer, Sir Donald Acheson.

Before the Public Inquiry on the Stanley Royd episode had had the opportunity to report, a further hospital-associated outbreak had given similar cause for concern. In April 1985 a number of patients attending the outpatient department, or admitted as inpatients, at the new Stafford District General Hospital were unwittingly exposed to an aerosol containing virulent *Legionella pneumophilia* organisms emanating from the hospital's cooling tower. A total of 68 confirmed cases of Legionnaires' disease were subsequently treated in hospital with 22 deaths. A further 35 cases were suspected cases. All these patients had visited the hospital during April 1985. Nearly one third of hospital staff were also shown to have *Legionella* antibodies and some of these demonstrated "influenza-like" illnesses (O'Mahony et al. 1990). The Committee of Inquiry on this outbreak not only made recommendations regarding the engineering safety aspects of cooling towers of this sort but also raised doubts about the competence of MOsEH in dealing with outbreaks of infection (Department of Health and Social Security 1986b). This last point clearly added weight to the need for the Chief Medical Officer's Committee to debate the role of the specialty of community medicine within the "public health function."

The outcome of the Acheson Committee's deliberations was a report of major significance, *Public Health in England* (1988), usually referred to as the Acheson Report, which went far beyond the issue of communicable disease control, and the implementation of which gave health authorities, for the first time, the responsibilities of assessing the health needs of their population and of meeting these needs. A Director of Public Health (DPH) was to be appointed to advise on the discharge of these responsibilities. Generally in practice, at least initially, the existing DMO simply took on the additional responsibilities. A particularly interesting inclusion in the DPH's duties was the preparation and publication of an Annual Report on the health of the District's population. Annual Reports were not, of course, new in the evolution of public health systems. The preparation of such a report had been a formal responsibility of the Medical Officer of Health until this requirement lapsed with the coming to an end of the post itself in 1974. This new, post-Acheson, Annual Report clearly had the potential to be more influential as it was to be an integral component of the health authority's planning cycle and was also to represent a source of information for local authorities and other local bodies on local health issues . The Department of Health itself produced some guidance on content by producing a series of publications entitled *Public Health Common Data Set* (1989), assembling in one place demographic, morbidity, and mortality information, including cancer registrations and congenital malformations relevant to each District.

But how the Annual Report was to be *perceived* was very important. Data-handling staff might semi-dismissively use expressions such as "just the usual annual stats stuff" but such a perception would almost certainly have been a turn-off for most people. Accordingly it was important for the DPH to use the relevant local data to form the basis of a document which would, ideally, interpret the local findings, comment on them, draw conclusions from them, and finally make recommendations which would make sense to the readership. It might even lead to appropriate action! The formal requirement for each DPH to produce an Annual Report was to operate from October 1990, covering the previous year, but my colleagues and I in the Department of Public Health Medicine in Coventry decided to prepare an informal one for the year 1988. Because of the "unofficial" status of the latter, no resources were allocated for this project and so its enthusiastic authors used every form of ingenuity to assemble the material, prepare illustrations etc., where necessary calling in favours from well-funded organisations to help to produce an effective and professional-looking publication. The entire text was meticulously typed on a goodwill basis by my secretary.

It certainly turned out to be an eye-catching document. The cover was a folder which, when opened out, was shown to be a map of Coventry which was designed to be overlaid by a series of eight transparency maps in an attempt to relate e.g. unemployment rates by Electoral wards, childhood accidents by Postcode Area, immunisation uptake by neighbourhood areas, number of years lost under the age of 75 by Electoral ward etc. These overlay maps, placed one on another, could demonstrate, for example, that high unemployment was closely correlated to a high number of years of life lost, and that there was an inverse relationship between immunisation and fertility rates, suggesting that mothers with large families might be finding it difficult to attend immunisation sessions. The chapter titles, similarly, were meant to catch one's attention. Instead of *Demography* there was *Peoples and Places,* for *Mortality Data* there was *Death in Coventry*, and one headed *Lifestyles* was based on a Regionally organised random sample survey of the local population's eating, drinking, smoking and exercising habits. A chapter entitled *Fevers* replaced the more traditional *Infectious Diseases* and showed, amongst other things, that the death rate from tuberculosis was inordinately high, a finding that understandably caused the health authority members considerable discomfort but had the positive effect of leading to a demand for even more intensive preventive and control action to combat this disease (Pollock 1989). [Six years later the "Coventry team," by that time each member having moved on, had a chapter entitled "*How to write—and use—the Annual Report of the Director of Public Health*" (Binysh et al. 1995) included in the British Medical Journal's "How to do it" series. In fact, even 3 years prior to the publication of the Acheson Report, Coventry had already identified the value of a report on the health of its population. In 1985, the Department of Public Health Medicine, having been strengthened by the recruitment of enthusiastic young trainees who had radical ideas about public health's role, produced a report entitled *The Health of Coventry* (Binysh et al. 1985) which had a profound impact locally. This became the subject of a major local conference, bringing together not only health professional but also those representing the environment, education, housing, employment, the food industry, the water company and the police, because of the significant influences which these services have on our health. The conference was filmed and the video has been used for training purposes both in this country and Montreal, Canada.]

The Acheson Report gave particular attention to the unsatisfactory nature of the MOEH appointment. It expressed the belief that this post, straddling uncomfortably between health and local authorities, had proved unsatisfactory in practice and should be abolished. The title of the replacement post, likely to be from a background of public health medicine, medical microbiology or clinical infectious disease, caused some debate. The first suggestion was "District Control of Infection Officer," but when this was shortened to DCIO and soon light-heartedly referred to as "DC Ten" (the most popular charter holiday jet of the period) this idea was dropped. Similarly the "Medical Officer for Communicable Disease Control" initials—MOCDC—soon referred to as "Mock Doc" were clearly not going to do anything to improve the status of the post! Eventually the title of Consultant in Communicable Disease Control (CCDC) was adopted and this individual was to have *executive responsibility for the surveillance, prevention and control of communicable disease and infection at local, i.e. District Health Authority, level.*

The outcome of this reappraisal, the organisational framework with the CCDC at its heart, represented what was felt to be an appropriate arrangement within the new management structure of the NHS. The "consultant" part of the CCDC title was important for the purposes of according the correct status to the role, the bureaucratic term "officer" (as in MOEH) having been left behind. The Acheson Committee's view was that only if the individual focused exclusively on the surveillance, prevention and control of communicable disease and infection would he or she be accepted as a genuine specialist both within and outside the NHS. Perhaps paradoxically (but understandably) the Committee was equally concerned that the CCDC needed to operate within a "managed situation" of accountability (Cunningham D, 1990, Personal communication. Interview with author. Department of Health, London, 21st December 1990), to minimise the possibility of repetition of incidents such as Stanley Royd and Stafford.

At the time of the Government's 1968 Green Paper on health service reorganisation, described in Chap. 5, the law on the control of communicable disease had seemed rather dated, and this situation still prevailed in 1988 when the Acheson Committee was considering this aspect of the public health function. For example, some of the legal provisions covered such archaic issues as the handling of library books, the keeping of common lodging houses, and the restriction of wakes. In fact, to quote from the Committee's deliberations:

> ....There was widespread uncertainty about the precise provisions of the law, and guidance issued by the DHSS to health authorities and local authorities in 1973, for example whether responsibility for the control of communicable diseases, other than notifiable infections and food poisoning, rested with the health authority or local authority. The law needed to be clarified.

The Committee accepted that the lack of clarity about the roles and responsibilities in this field derived from the complexity of out-dated legislation and from misunderstanding about its interpretation. It was acknowledged that the Public Health Acts comprised a complex body of legislation, stretching back for more than a century, which did not seek to codify the *responsibilities* of authorities in respect of communicable disease but rather conferred certain reserve *powers* which might be necessary. Accordingly, one of the Acheson Report's key recommendations was that there should be a revision of the Public Health (Control of Disease) Act 1984 with a view to producing a more up-to-date and relevant legislative backing to the control of communicable disease and infection. To aid this revision, the Department of Health produced in 1989 a consultative document, *Review of Law on Infectious Disease Control* (Department of Health 1989) which had wide circulation but, even now in 2011, no new legislation for this purpose has yet appeared on the Statute Book! Informal soundings from the Department of Health at the time revealed that "the subject never quite got to the top of the priority list—there was always something more important." A secondary view, as far as lack of clarity was concerned, seemed to be along the lines of "we expect you chaps to work out these things sensibly." Accordingly, the application of formal measures for the control of communicable disease in England rests on the legislation which is extant, namely the Public Health (Control of Disease) Act 1984 and the Public Health (Infectious Diseases) Regulations 1988.

The above Act and Regulations did at least give the MOEH (and subsequently the CCDC) the authority to, for example, receive reports of notifiable infectious diseases, exclude an infectious child from school, require an infectious individual to discontinue work, require the medical examination of an individual or group of individuals, or require the admission of an infectious person to hospital and if necessary detention there. Legal safeguards ensure that no individual is deprived of his or her liberty unless it is absolutely necessary to prevent spread of infection. *Compulsory* admission to, and detention in, hospital to prevent spread of infection is an extremely rare event. I only once found it necessary to invoke this in nearly four decades of public health practice, a middle-aged man with infectious pulmonary tuberculosis who refused to take the relevant drugs and insisted on having close contact with young children in his neighbourhood.

Curiously enough, almost certainly because of an administrative oversight, the legislation did *not* give the MOEH/CCDC the authority to enforce surveillance of contacts, or isolation at home (Button J, 1999, Public health legal information unit, Matlock, Derbyshire. Personal communication. Telephone conversation 11th

January 1999). As I mentioned in Chap. 5, I was not actually aware of the *absence* of such authority when I enforced home isolation and surveillance of contacts in the case of the suspected case of smallpox in Coventry in April 1973; fortunately, on that occasion, the family members had given their informed consent to these restrictions and cheerfully complied in all respects!

The use of the law to prevent the spread of HIV infection has been even less straightforward. Musto (1991) has expressed the view that the fear of diseases such as HIV arises not just because of the effects of the virus itself but also from a consideration of the types of individuals who are likely to be predisposed to this kind of infection. In fact, in England, a very small number of individuals *have* been successfully prosecuted for "recklessly inflicting grievous bodily harm" on their sexual partners, under the Offences Against the Person Act of 1861 (Coker 2006). It is somewhat surprisingly that this is the only piece of legislation which can be invoked in these circumstances, and can presumably be justified only in highly unusual circumstances where it is felt that an individual needs to be detained for the protection of others. One might also assume that the media publicity associated with such cases would discourage similar behaviour.

Interestingly, in 1988, the question of control of infection in *hospitals* was being looked at quite separately from the considerations of the Acheson Committee, although in a sense in parallel with them. Experience in the United States had shown that the existence of hospital infection control teams greatly reduced infection rates in these establishments. A working group set up jointly by the Department of Health and Social Security and the Public Health Laboratory Service produced its guidance document *Hospital Infection Control* ,(usually referred to as the Cooke Report as it had been chaired by Professor Mary Cooke), which dealt with the management arrangements required for this purpose including the establishment of Hospital Infection Control Committees and Teams and the appointment of Infection Control Doctors and Nurses in all hospitals providing acute services. It was reassuring to note the recommendation that the team should include the MOEH among its members, although the topic of hospital infection control arrangements had received scant reciprocal attention in the Acheson Report itself (BMJ Editorial 1989). This guidance also advised on the actual management of outbreaks in hospital and the impact on the hospital of community outbreaks. [Seven years later it was necessary to update this guidance in the light of the many changes which had occurred, including the role of the CCDC post, and the developments in medical practice which had led to shorter stays in hospital for many patients so that hospital-acquired infections might now well present initially in the community (Department of Health/Public Health Laboratory Service 1995).]

Chapter 7
No Lasting Stability

In as much as the main reason for the establishment of the 1986 *Public Health Enquiry* was the identification of problems concerned with the control of communicable disease, it was important to ensure that its recommendations were being implemented. By a curious set of coincidences, I found myself almost immediately deeply involved in many of the activities flowing from the Government's acceptance of the recommendations. Having indicated my intention to take premature retirement from Coventry Health Authority in 1990 in order to develop my teaching activities at Warwick University, where I had been a visiting senior lecturer in community medicine for 10 years, I found that the fact that I was immediately available for part-time work led to a number of interesting invitations from a variety of organisations all of which were focused on one or other aspect of implementing the *Acheson* recommendations.

The first two approaches came simultaneously from the Director of CDSC, Dr Chris Bartlett, and Dr Deirdre Cunningham, Head of the Public Health Division at the Department of Health, who jointly recruited me essentially to carry out a survey of the 14 Regional Health Authorities in order to ascertain who would be discharging the duties of CCDC in each district, the professional background of each post holder and what specific training needs might be identified for the competent discharge of the relevant duties. These regional visits also would provide the opportunity to identify those trainees (mainly in public health medicine and medical microbiology) who might be keen to become CCDCs, and which in turn might give an indication of the need for training programmes that could be provided by universities or other educational establishments (Department of Health 1990). The third approach was more local. As it was my intention to continue to reside in the West Midlands, the Regional Medical Officer, Dr Michael Harrison, suggested that I should not neglect my "home" Region and therefore I gladly also accepted his invitation to take on the part-time role of coordinator of training programmes in communicable disease control for the West Midlands. These three interlocking sets of duties, none of which in itself was too demanding or time-consuming, produced the amusing result that, retiring from Coventry HA on the 31st May 1990, I recommenced work on the

G. Pollock, *An Epidemiological Odyssey: The Evolution of Communicable Disease Control*, DOI 10.1007/978-94-007-3998-7_7,

following day, operating from three separate locations considerable distances apart. As this was at a time when mobile telephones were not very common, my wife generously provided the coordinating link from our Coventry home.

At the same time, a steering group chaired by Professor David Miller of St Mary's Hospital was set up by the Faculty of Public Health Medicine, the Royal College of Pathologists and the Royal College of Physicians to examine the existing educational facilities which might contribute to the relevant training programmes. It was thought helpful for a small sub-group to carry out the detailed work on behalf of the steering group and I readily undertook to be its convenor; it was chaired initially by Professor Raj Bhopal of Newcastle University and subsequently by myself. The task took 4 years and the outcome was the report *Training for the CCDC Role* (Pollock et al. 1994), published by the (then) Faculty of Public Health Medicine in London.

It soon became apparent that England's response to the Acheson Report, during the first half of the 1990s, was far-reaching and in some depth. There was a strongly perceived need for people to be protected against communicable diseases and, unlike some other good ideas emanating from national committees from time to time, action did in fact follow. Two fields of practice within medicine were clearly able to make the major contribution, namely public health medicine/epidemiology and medical microbiology. Although the specialty of clinical infectious diseases had "equal rights" in this field it was found, in practice, that very few of these physicians applied for CCDC posts although the Royal College of Physicians was strongly represented on the steering group on training referred to above. (It would be idle to try to hide the fact that there was a measure of "healthy rivalry" between the epidemiologists and the microbiologists at this time but all committees or groups tended to ensure that both specialties had equal representation. A major joint conference held in June 1990, with a view to giving a full airing to these issues, was so well subscribed that the main hall of the Royal Institute of British Architects had to be hired to accommodate all those attending. An epidemiologist chaired the morning session and a microbiologist the afternoon one; much of the discussion was of the kind usually referred to as "full, frank and useful.")

A further feature of the situation during this period was that the country became much more outward-looking with regard to understanding these problems, showing greater interest in how other nations were tackling them. As one example of this development, in June 1991 I was sent by Dr Harrison to CDC Atlanta, in order to gain a general picture of how the USA was responding to the threats and specifically to learn about the relatively new computerised surveillance system known as *Epi-Info* and to bring back its software so that it could be introduced locally. In this connection, I was allowed to train at CDC alongside the state epidemiologists, being given the light-hearted title of "honorary state epidemiologist." The reverse of this situation also applied; other countries were interested in what we were doing, and I was fortunate enough to have the experience of being invited to take part in seminars on the events in England in places as far apart as UCLA, the Oklahoma State Health Department and the University of Helsinki.

Back in England, however, it was felt that the special situation of Greater London deserved particular consideration, taking into account the fact that many people might live in one part of the metropolis, work in quite a different part, and engage in social activities (including eating out) in a variety of locations relatively remote from both home and work. Given also that many thousands arrive in the capital each day by air, rail and road, it was clear that communicable disease surveillance and control were of paramount importance. Accordingly in 1993 I was commissioned jointly by the four Thames Regional Health Authorities to examine the situation across Greater London—comprising 41 separate District Health Authorities, each with its own CCDC—and report accordingly. The four Regional Directors of Public Health kindly arranged a series of appointments in Central London for me to meet the CCDCs and take evidence from them. (Without such an arrangement the project would probably have proved impracticable within a reasonable time-frame.) The main outcome of the study was the acknowledgement of the need for shared surveillance data across Greater London (Pollock 1993) and accordingly a Pan-London Change Management Group was set up to take this forward. As a result, in 1994, the London Communicable Disease Surveillance Project came into being, funded jointly by the four Thames Regions and the Department of Health and based at CDSC Colindale and with its own monthly publication, the *Thames Monitor*. [Achieving this outcome required thoughtfulness and sensitivity. Individual District CCDCs, quite understandably, felt that their District data belonged to *them*—they had collected it and they would be utilising it. However a compromise was readily reached by which District CCDCs would submit their data for a shared surveillance base covering Greater London on the clear understanding that all control activities within a District would remain *their* responsibility.]

But what was actually happening in England, *in terms of communicable diseases themselves,* in the wake of the Acheson Report? I had some indication of one issue at my first meeting with Dr Harrison on taking up my part-time duties at the West Midlands RHA in June 1990, when he apologised for the tuna sandwiches instead of the usual corned beef ones offered, explaining that this was an instruction from the Authority's Chairman; in the latter's words, up to that point there had been no evidence of any condition that might be referred to as "mad tuna disease!" Certainly at that time there was considerable public anxiety that the cattle disease *bovine spongiform encephalopathy* (BSE) —so-called "mad cow disease"—might have been spread to humans, and in that year a national surveillance unit had in fact been set up in Edinburgh to monitor this possibility. The justification for this concern was that the evidence suggested that BSE in cattle had been caused by their being fed meat and bone meal from carcases of sheep suffering from *scrapie*, and therefore that the infection might cross the species barrier once more and infect humans who had eaten beef (Kimberlin and Walker 1989). The widespread publicity which this matter had received altered the dietary habits of large numbers of people and food retailers were quick to respond by replacing beef, for example in pies, by other meats such as chicken. In Scotland, the well-known small round individual meat pies, an inexpensive local delicacy, were frequently filled with macaroni cheese instead. The situation even caused me a moment of minor personal embarrassment when my mother, at that time in her early 90s, insisted that it was my duty to instruct the staff of the residential home in which she was then living not to serve beef to any resident!

A condition known as *Creutzfeldt-Jacob Disease* (CJD), a form of rapidly progressive encephalopathy affecting older people, had for many years been known to exist (Department of Health 1995). But in 1996 the Edinburgh unit began to receive notifications of a similar clinical syndrome affecting much younger persons and running a more protracted course. Investigation led to the conclusion that in these cases consumption of infected beef had taken place before 1988, when a ban on feeding the suspected material to cattle had been introduced. This new syndrome, quickly given the name *new variant CJD* (vCJD), was therefore regarded as the consequence of being exposed to the infected meat. In 1997 it was concluded that the agent which causes vCJD in human beings was the same as that which causes BSE in cattle (Department of Health 1997). This represented a bitter irony as in 1990 the Department of Health, on the basis of professional advice, had issued a statement via the Chief Medical Officer, Sir Donald Acheson himself, that "if there were any hazard for man from oral ingestion of beef or beef products, the risk would be very small indeed" (Department of Health 1990). Surveillance by the Edinburgh unit has continued and at the time of writing (October 2011) 1,647 deaths from vCJD had been notified. Various aspects of medical, surgical and dental practice have had to be modified in the light of this risk of contamination by blood or blood products. A great step forward was taken in February 2011 when the MRC Prion Unit at University College London announced that its scientists had developed the world's first reliable blood test for vCJD. This should greatly aid diagnosis, and also allow screening and identification of carriers with great significance for ensuring the safety of blood transfusion (Edgeworth et al. 2011).

Another communicable disease was being recognised as a public health problem about this time—Hepatitis C. Although since the 1970s microbiologists had been aware of a further form of hepatitis which they were referring to as "non-A, non-B" it was not until April 1989 that the responsible virus was discovered and named Hepatitis C and even in the following year reliable tests for use on a routine basis were only just becoming available (Department of Health 1990). The virus is spread by blood-to-blood contact and in England the majority of infections are spread by sharing of needles and other "equipment" by injecting drug misusers. Sexual transmission is not considered common and specific screening of blood and blood products has cut across that particular path of transmission. The sinister aspect of hepatitis C infection is that the early stages are usually symptomless but, without treatment, about 85% go on to develop a chronic infection, with the risk of cirrhosis and a form of liver cancer. Routine screening of blood donations for anti-HCV (Hepatitis C virus) began on 1st September 1991 (Department of Health 1991).

It is interesting to note that the coming into being of the CCDC post, as an important recommendation of the Acheson Report, could hardly have made much difference with regard to the incidence of the above two infections in the early stages as they are both relatively "silent" chronic infections without readily identifiable symptoms of onset. On the other hand, both conditions obviously called for surveillance data as backcloth to measures of prevention and control, including a major component of health education.

The next communicable disease episode, however, could not have presented a greater contrast. The pandemic of *Severe Acute Respiratory Syndrome* (SARS), a pneumonia-like infection by a new member of the coronavirus family (World Health Organisation 2003a), was indeed severe and acute, the disease having an incubation period of no more than 10 days and a case-fatality rate of just under 10%. As coronaviruses are important pathogens of mammals and birds it was considered that these might have constituted the origin of the human infection (Fouchier et al. 2003). Although England did not have many suspected cases, it would be totally false to suggest that the country was not very heavily involved for a period of a few months. In fact, it would be fair to state that most countries in the world had their public health prevention and control systems tested to the hilt by this phenomenon, as the following account shows.

It is highly probable that the pandemic began in Guangdong Province, China, in November 2002 when a farmer was admitted to a local hospital—The First People's Hospital at Foshan—and died. It is a matter of note that studies of samples of wild animals sold as food in the local market in Guangdong in May 2003 revealed that the SARS coronavirus could be isolated from palm civets (Wenhui et al. 2006). No notification was made to WHO by the Chinese Health Authorities at the time but Canada's component of the WHO's Global Outbreak and Alert Response Network picked up reports of a "flu outbreak" in China on 27 November 2002 (Heymann and Rodier 2004).

In February 2003 an American businessman was taken off a China to Singapore flight at Hanoi, Vietnam, because of what appeared to be a serious form of pneumonia. He died in hospital there and a number of medical staff who had treated him also became ill with the same disease in spite of routine hospital infection control measures. Particularly tragically, the doctor there who identified the condition and alerted WHO was himself fatally affected. This episode, understandably, received much media publicity and on 12 March 2003 WHO issued a global alert. Local transmission of the condition now known as "SARS" occurred within Canada, the United States, Ulan Bator, the Philippines, Taiwan, Vietnam and Hong Kong, in addition to spreading within many parts of China itself. Quarantine of contacts and closure of schools were introduced in many affected countries in an attempt to control further spread of SARS. On 27 March, WHO recommended screening of airline passengers for symptoms of the condition (World Health Organisation 2003b), and on 23 April advised against all but essential travel to Toronto. (This latter recommendation caused me a slight degree of apprehension as, just at that point, an old school friend emailed me from Toronto asking me to meet him at Aberdeen Airport as he was aware that I would be spending a few days there at the time of his visit. As he didn't refer to SARS, I felt too embarrassed to raise the subject but heartily wished that he were coming from some other part of the globe, such was the fear, especially among doctors, of the infectiousness and lethal potential of the condition!)

The numbers involved globally were very high indeed. Between November 2002 and July 2003 there were 8,096 known cases with 774 deaths. England escaped comparatively lightly with just four suspected cases (i.e. those which met the agreed case definition), the first two having recently returned from Hong Kong and Taiwan respectively, although there was reasonably good evidence of a number of further infections which did not meet the suspect or probable case definition and, fortunately, were probably of minimal infectiousness (Nicoll A, 2003, Personal communication. Letter to author, 3rd November 2003).

As was mentioned earlier, although England was only minimally involved in terms of the number of suspected cases, this does not mean that the country did not play a major part in the unprecedented degree of international collaboration which the pandemic brought about, in addition to responding vigorously internally at national, regional and local level. Chapter 6 explained in detail how an excellent surveillance system had been set up and this proved its value throughout this episode in the way in which suspected cases and their contacts were promptly and effectively dealt with. The national reference laboratory at Colindale played a major role in this. The system demonstrated considerable "surge capacity" to deal with the additional pressures but only at the expense of some staff having to be diverted from their usual tasks. [The question of surge capacity for communicable disease control, especially at local level, has represented a matter of major concern since the abolition of the post of Medical Officer of Health in 1974. The point is one of such fundamental importance that it is dealt with in some detail in Chap. 8.]

The situation in England was made more challenging by the fact that the pandemic occurred at a time of great reorganisation in the services provided for communicable disease control. A major change was the establishment of the Health Protection Agency (HPA) on 1 April 2003—in the middle of the whole episode—bringing into one central Agency a number of health protection bodies including the PHLS and incorporating local CCDCs into its local health protection teams. From that point onwards, the HPA coordinated the operational public health response. This response included an on-going process of contingency planning in the belief that SARS might not have "gone away" (Harper 2004). This view, i.e. the need to avoid any complacency, was also expressed by the then Director of the PHLS Communicable Disease Control Centre, Professor Angus Nicoll, who felt that one of the factors which had allowed England to get its preparations in place in good time was the experience gained in such places as Hong Kong and Canada which had been among the countries earliest affected (Nicoll A, 2003, Personal communication. Letter to author, 3rd November 2003).

The background to the creation of the HPA was as follows. A 2002 Government report, *Getting Ahead of the Curve: a strategy for combating infectious diseases (including other aspects of health protection)*, declared the intention to create a new Health Protection Agency which would provide a more integrated approach to all aspects of health protection: against infectious diseases, together with chemical and radiological hazards. The new Agency was therefore to absorb the existing functions of the PHLS (including its Communicable Disease Surveillance Centre), the Centre for Applied Microbiological Research, the National Focus for Chemical Incidents, and the National Radiological Protection Board. As mentioned above, the new Agency became operational on I April 2003 when the PHLS was already heavily engaged in dealing with the national response to the SARS pandemic—"a baptism of fire for the entire Agency," as it was described (Harper 2004).

The role of the Agency is to identify and respond to health hazards and emergencies caused by infectious disease, hazardous chemicals, poisons or radiation. It works at international, national, regional and local levels. Although set up by the Government, the Agency is independent and provides whatever advice and information is necessary to protect people's health. Local and Regional Agency services work alongside the NHS. In addition to the Centre for Infection (which absorbed the functions of the PHLS, including its Communicable Disease Control Centre), there are Centres for Emergency Preparedness and Response, Radiation, Chemical and Environmental Hazards, and the National Institute for Biological Standards and Controls. The Centre for Infections at Colindale is the base for national communicable disease surveillance and specialist microbiology (Health Protection Agency website 2010a).

It was not very long after the end of the SARS episode that concern began to be focused on the possibility of another pandemic—influenza. Ever since the first pandemic of AH1N1 infection in 1918/1919, referred to as "Spanish influenza," there had been fears of a further world-wide recurrence of this or a similar virus. But it was not until 1957 that it appeared that such fears might be justified when the AH2N2 variant emerged, referred to as "Asian influenza" because of its origin in the Far East in May of that year. Cases began to occur in England as early as the following month and during the winter of 1957/1958 there were approximately 50,000 influenza-related deaths (Donaldson and Scally 2009). I remember the situation well as a vaccine was offered from November 1957. My fiancée and I had the first of the two doses, but the second was due only a few days before we were due to be married and so we declined the follow-up, not wishing to be indisposed on our honeymoon!

A third pandemic began in 1968, yet again in the Far East, and was referred to as Hong Kong influenza (or, as the media called it, "Mao flu," implying perhaps a political in additional to an epidemiological threat!). The virus on this occasion was AH3N2. I also recall this episode vividly but for a very different reason: in my capacity of Deputy Medical Officer of Health of the City of Coventry, I had to first convince the City Council's Finance Committee of the necessity to release funds to purchase the relevant vaccine and then to persuade those in the front-line community and public services of the advisability of being vaccinated. This meant not only the doctors, health visitors, district nurses and midwives, but also many others such as those who manned the City's buses, the Fire and Rescue Services. I have clear memories of many busy evenings in the Central Fire Station's main hall, vaccinating large groups as they came off duty or shift. In the event, this particular epidemic was not quite as serious as might have been expected, at least as far as England was concerned.

A "false alarm" occurred in 1976 in the United States. In January of that year a virus identified as "swine flu," isolated from four sick Army recruits at Fort Dix, New Jersey was thought to be similar to the AH1N1 organism responsible for the 1918 pandemic. By March, CDC Atlanta and he United States Public Health Service had been able to persuade President Ford to approve funds of $135 million for the preparation of an effective vaccine to be ready for mass use by October. Within 10 weeks almost 50 million Americans had been vaccinated. Unfortunately, by mid-December, a causal relationship had been identified between the vaccine and a small number of cases of Guillain-Barré paralysis and, as there had been no further cases of "swine flu" since the original four, the vaccination campaign was suspended (Mullan 1989).

Obviously, after three pandemics in just half a century, epidemiologists were convinced that it would be only a matter of time before the next threat appeared and the Department of Health in London continued to develop contingency plans for such an event. In fact, in the Annual Report of the Chief Medical Officer for 2005, he stated: "*When the influenza pandemic arrives, health care facilities will be under enormous pressure and will need to be targeted at those most in need. The pandemic will pose a unique challenge to NHS emergency planning in the modern era. Clear national policies and strong, well-rehearsed local plans will be the keys to mitigating its effects.*"

It had been felt that the danger signals for a fourth pandemic were emerging when, towards the end of 2003, just a few months after the end of the SARS episode, cases of AH5N1 influenza were reported in Vietnam and China with a number of deaths, all in individuals who were working closely with poultry, and the terms Avian Influenza and "bird flu" came Into general use. (Originally it had been considered that Avian influenza did not normally infect species other than birds and pigs but there had been one episode in Hong Kong in 1997 in which 18 persons had been infected, with six deaths. On epidemiological grounds the virus had spread directly from birds to humans and this was confirmed by genetic studies.) One of the outbreaks in late 2003 was reported in a letter from Chinese scientists to the June 2004 issue of the New England Journal of Medicine and the Chinese Health Ministry informed WHO of the confirmation of this by laboratory tests. Although there was no convincing evidence that human to human spread was happening—all the cases had had very close contact with poultry—the memory of SARS was sufficiently recent to cause a certain amount of global anxiety; epidemiologists world-wide were expressing fears that the virus might mutate into a form which could allow human to human transmission. What actually transpired was that AH5N1 infections appeared to smoulder on, with poultry-associated cases and deaths mainly in the Far East. The media always seemed to be hinting that a human pandemic might be imminent and much publicity was given to the only two anti-virals which were considered to have some action against the virus, *Tamiflu* and *Relenza.* Aware of the anxieties being quietly expressed in the autumn of 2005 by some of my epidemiology colleagues, I gave way to family pressure and obtained a supply of *Tamiflu* and a box of face masks which, fortunately, never had to be used.

In contrast to Avian Influenza, so-called "Swine Influenza" when it arrived in April 2009 seemed, on the face of it, to present a real threat to humans. This was a global outbreak of a new strain of AH1N1 influenza virus which appeared to have resulted when a previous triple reassortment of bird, pig and human influenza viruses further combined with a Eurasian pig influenza (Hellerman 2009). The outbreak began in Veracruz, Mexico but continued to spread globally. The case-fatality rate appeared high initially but this was later put in perspective as the view generally developed that many milder cases had not come within any medical ambit and that the actual case denominator was very much larger than had originally been realised.

In June 2009 both WHO and CDC Atlanta declared this outbreak a pandemic. In spite of its unofficial label, the AH1N1 infection was not spread by eating pork, but from person to person by droplet spray.

The first cases in England were reported on the 27th April 2009. Children were most affected and adults over 50 years of age had much lower attack rates. There were two waves of activity separated by the closure of schools over the summer, the first in mid/late July 2009 and the second peaking in mid-October 2009. The West Midlands and the London area were most affected in the early stages. The case-fatality rate was estimated to be 0.04%, most deaths being in persons under the age of 65 years. Anti-viral drugs were offered to those with suggestive symptoms and these significantly reduced the length of the illness. They were also valuable in reducing the incidence of secondary cases in household contacts. A vaccine programme was begun in October 2009 initially for front-line health care workers, pregnant women, and those aged between 6 months and 65 years who were in the defined clinical at-risk groups. From December 2009 the vaccine was also offered to healthy children between 6 months and 5 years of age (Health Protection Agency Website 2010b). The pandemic began to taper off in November 2009 and by May 2010 the number of cases was in steep decline. On August 10th 2010, WHO declared that the pandemic was over.

The pandemic presented critical emergency planning, response and recovery challenges at both national and local levels. The public health response required the assessment of hundreds of thousands of cases nationally, the delivery of enormous quantities of anti-viral medicines and a massive vaccination programme, while planning for the anticipated loss of key services and staff through illness. Throughout the progress of the pandemic both public and medical perceptions shifted from near panic to indifference as all struggled to respond to changing and sometimes conflicting public communications. In Sandwell, West Midlands, for example, the scale of the required response regarding both anti-virals and vaccination meant that large numbers of staff of the Primary Health Care Trust had to be rapidly redeployed from their normal duties, being joined by staff of the Local Authority and other local bodies in developments which rapidly took on a "febrile" tempo (Saunders 2011).

Unfortunately the infection re-emerged just before Christmas 2010, leaving doctors puzzled, but after seeming to settle down, as Watson and Pebody (2011) have pointed out, the recent 2010/2011 seasonal activity in the UK and other European countries has shown that the threat of pandemic infection has not disappeared. The whole episode has not passed without a certain amount of critical comment. For example, the European Parliament in January 2011 launched a strong attack on the World Health Organisation's handling of the situation by its (alleged) distortion of the term "pandemic" and setting off a world-wide false alarm and thus giving rise to disproportionate public health decisions by European Union countries (Watson 2011).

It is with some regret that I have to end this continuous narrative on a note of considerable uncertainty with regard to the future arrangements for the prevention and control of communicable diseases in England. The new Coalition Government, elected in May 2010, has declared its intention, in a White Paper *Equity and*

Excellence: Liberating the NHS, followed by the Health and Social Care Bill (at present before Parliament), to undertake a radical reform of the NHS, abolishing the existing management structures at both strategic and local levels and making general practitioner consortia responsible for commissioning the majority of health services for their local communities. Commissioning is intended to be based on knowledge of local needs, thus theoretically avoiding previous problems with over-commissioning of services and subsequent financial waste (Vaid 2010).

The Government has also made it clear, in a further White Paper, *Healthy Lives, Healthy People*, that it intends to dismantle the HPA and place the responsibility for the majority of public health services on Local Authorities, to which Directors of Public Health are now to be accountable. (As an ex-Medical Officer of Health, accountable at the time to Coventry City Council, I cannot but be reminded of the situation prior to April 1974. *Plus ça change….*!)The rationale behind this change is that it is believed that such a service will give more power to local people over their health in tackling such problems as obesity, alcohol dependence, smoking, sexually-transmitted infections, and poor mental health. Furthermore, the expectation is that Directors of Public Health will be able to champion cooperation at local level so that health issues are considered alongside services such as housing, transport and education, thus creating an environment conducive to healthy choices. The exercise of such choices will clearly be important as the Government has made it clear that it will "stay out" of people's everyday lives wherever possible, and instead will "nudge" people in the direction of choosing healthily. There is currently much professional and public discussion concerning the meaning of this word (new, in this context!) At a national level, a new core public health service—*Public Health England*—is to combine experts from public health bodies such as the Health Protection Agency and the National Treatment Agency as a part of the Department of Health itself. *Public Health England* will actually be accountable to the Head of the Civil Service—and not to the Chief Medical Officer; this means that, for the first time, the CMO will not be responsible for public health in England (Field 2011), a somewhat paradoxical situation as the CMO's Annual Report was traditionally entitled *On The State Of The Public Health*. The Local Health Protection Units, broadly similar to those currently provided by the Health Protection Agency, are now to operate within its framework. It is presumed that CCDCs will work within these Units. *Public Health England* is also to be the appointing agency for Director of Public Health posts and the national source of professional support to such posts in their Local Authority setting.

Chapter 8
Tailpiece

People always seem to have had a particular fear of infectious diseases. There are many possible reasons for this. The fact that the causative agents are invisible—like ionising radiation—must surely be one, and the very brevity of the incubation period of many fevers could provoke further anxiety, especially if an outbreak appears to be running wildfire within a local community, individuals wondering "who's next?" There can also be the implied disapproval of some aspect of someone's lifestyle, such as an assumption of unhygienic living conditions or perhaps sexual indiscretion. This anxiety is not necessarily confined to individuals. Families may wish to conceal the fact that a member has a disease such as tuberculosis, for example, for fear of being kept at a distance by neighbours. Even governments may feel that they have reason to conceal the nature or extent of a particular outbreak and consequently fail to notify the World Health Organisation for inclusion in its Weekly Epidemiological Bulletin.

Against this background, what evidence is there of man's attempts to combat these diseases? And to what extent have such attempts required organised action by whatever form of society prevailed at the time? Certainly in earliest times, group or societal action would appear to be the more prominent, although this could simply mean that the actions of individuals were likely to go unrecorded, whereas societies have tended to leave their mark, whether or not intentionally. There are, of course, a small number of exceptions: the personal observations of Sushruta, Hippocrates, Varro and Bede, and of course later on Fracastoro, for example, represented remarkable individual contributions to understanding the behaviour of infectious diseases, almost certainly more than they themselves realised.

However one of the most surprising things is just how long it took for mankind to realise that certain diseases *were*, in fact, communicable. One would have thought that Hippocrates would have accepted this concept totally by virtue of the fact that his approach to the study of "epidemics" was governed essentially by observation and deduction. Instead he favoured the inclusion of the ideas of corrupt air, imbalance of the bodily humours, and the particular positions of the heavenly bodies. And although, in the first century BC, Marcus Varro had clearly described

G. Pollock, *An Epidemiological Odyssey: The Evolution of Communicable Disease Control*, DOI 10.1007/978-94-007-3998-7_8,

his theory of microbial life, this did not appear to have been deliberately incorporated into Roman thinking about action to promote health and prevent disease. By the nineteenth century, of course, the published findings of *individual* researchers such as Pasteur and Koch were far more prominent, available to guide those with responsibilities for the public health, although it can by no means assumed that health administrations were invariably inclined to try to take early advantage of the science. Even in twenty-first century England, examples of a medical research unit "feeding" information in the form of study reports as part of an on-going, integrated process for the purpose of guiding treatment strategies in a closely related hospital (as at Imperial College, London) are sufficiently uncommon to result in special comment in medical journals.

This account can in no sense represent a linear sequence. Sometimes many activities were going on in parallel in different countries, sometimes even in the same country, with little or no contact or communication between them. Microbiological research on the European Continent during the nineteenth century, for example, was running alongside public health legislative development in England, with little evidence that the latter was informed by the former. On occasions, two sets of activities might be pursuing separate paths, with quite different motivations, but unwittingly both contributing to the same outcome. As an illustration, in the 1830s and 1840s, the organisational response to cholera's penetration of the English quarantine arrangements was occurring at the same time as Chadwick's recommendations for the relief of poverty. Each was independent of the other—one concerned with community health protection, the other focusing on the utilitarian value of the economically active breadwinner—but together they contributed to the production of what might be regarded as the standard public health unit, a defined territory with responsibility for the control of infectious diseases locally and an appointed "public doctor" to be accountable for this. Lastly, quite fallacious beliefs could nevertheless lead to desirable outcomes: the sanitary engineering activities carried out to deal with the imagined hazards of the evil stench known as "miasma" fortuitously led to a major reduction in the incidence of gastrointestinal infections. And so, at least until the end of the nineteenth century, rather than a linear progression, the picture appears more like a mosaic with occasional interlinked strands.

There can be little doubt that the Roman presence in England for nearly three centuries must represent the first period in which an urban civilisation's impact on the country favoured a degree of protection against at least some infectious diseases. Even today, especially in the Developing World, clean drinking water is one of the two most important factors for such protection, (the other being routine childhood immunisation). What light was shed on the Dark Ages in England by Bede's eighth century writings simply revealed a country in which health-seeking behaviour influenced by scientific principles had been replaced by an exclusively religious view on the cause and treatment of disease. It took a further seven centuries, with the setting up of Caxton's printing press at Westminster, before there could once more begin to be opportunities for rediscovery of the shrewd observations of the Classical writers on, *inter alia*, communicable diseases.

A recurrent theme in this work has been the role of the state in the control of infectious diseases. This is considered justifiable as it has been intermittently a factor of significance for at least two and a half millennia, in fact since the Greek City States appointed municipal physicians to advise on the health of the population and the prevention of epidemics (Rosen 1958). The state has, of course, two roles: as a provider of services and as an enforcing authority. The latter is currently a live issue in England, as in other countries, mainly focusing on the tension between the restrictive power of the state, through the exercise of its laws, and the human rights of the individual. Perhaps the best current example is the question of the extent to which a prosecution can or should be brought against, or restrictions placed on, an individual who has knowingly and recklessly spread HIV infection. But as Gostin (2000) has put it: "*Does a coercive intervention truly reduce aggregate health risks, and what, if any, less intrusive interventions might reduce those risks as well or better*?

Additionally, from a totally different point of view, politicians attempting to minimise government expenditure on public services on the grounds of encouraging *individual* responsibility for one's own health and welfare may refer disparagingly to the so-called "nanny state," over-concerned with giving health advice to the nation, but a survey carried out in 2010 by *YouGov* showed that, for example,

82% of the public believe that alcohol manufacturers should have to print detailed information about the units of alcohol contained in the bottle or can,
81% that 2 h of sport per week should be made compulsory in schools,
78% that a simple at-a-glance food-labelling system should be introduced with clear information about levels of fat, sugar and salt,
74% that smoking in cars containing children should be banned (Faculty of Public Health 2010).

As was mentioned in Chap. 2, Porter (1999) makes the point that England was rather later than Continental Europe in instituting formal measures to control infectious diseases. However this is perhaps an oversimplification as although English towns did not have the autonomy or the precocity of (say) their Italian counterparts, and their governmental structures were much simpler, they did actually develop at roughly the same time, namely from the tenth to eleventh centuries and they certainly did have the authority to impose regulations by about 1,200, at least in the case of the larger towns. The volume and sophistication of regulation increased strongly thereafter, especially from the early fourteenth century (Watts J, 2010, Early mediaeval local authorities. Personal communication. Email to author 16th September 2010). In Coventry, for example, the year 1355 saw the replacement of authority of the Steward of the Lord of the Manor by that of the Mayor and Bailiffs of the "Leet," a court of justice having authority over a specified area and exercising legislative or bye-law-making activities (Smith 1945). Hence they were clearly in a position to exercise a degree of influence over the social devastation caused by the Black Death. In Coventry, however, this seems to have been more concerned with the disposition of property and the provision for dependants (Gooder 1998).

In as much as this chapter is attempting to provide an overview of the field, it would seem reasonable to think in terms of what "tools" the authorities in England have had at their disposal, and to consider what has been achieved, what is currently being dealt with, and what may have to be tackled in the future. These "tools" represent a wide variety of activities ranging from the simplest, based on everyday observation, such as isolation of infectious cases, to the more complex, depending on coordination of a number of separate processes each requiring scientific understanding, such as the importation, storage, handling and preparation of food, at each stage of which there exist opportunities for bacterial contamination. Obviously the simpler actions are the ones which were established early, whereas the more complex ones have had to await both scientific discoveries and the means of these being coordinated and integrated into daily living. Perhaps disappointingly, for those with neat and tidy minds, there appears to be no correlation between the level of achievement and the time when a particular control measure was introduced. For example, the eradication of smallpox had to await the ultimate success of the WHO vaccination campaign of the final quarter of the twentieth century; none of the earlier measures such as isolation of cases and fumigation of houses and possessions etc. could have achieved this. In addition to the roles and responsibilities of authorities, it may also be relevant (not least because of the current political emphasis on personal responsibility) to examine the extent to which individuals themselves can prevent or at least minimise the risk of infection, while also noting how some individuals may deny themselves or their children such protection for a variety of personal, cultural or religious reasons.

It is perhaps worth recalling the statement by Sir James Howie in 1970, referred to in Chap. 2: "*The best way to manage communicable diseases is to discover infections quickly and stop them from spreading*." As stated earlier, one could not wish for a more concise definition of the integration of *surveillance* and *control*. One simply needs to add *prevention* to complete the "package" of public health activities in this field. In fact, one could say that by far the most important recommendation of the 1988 Acheson Report, referred to in Chap. 6, and was that a named individual "should have executive responsibility for the ***surveillance***, ***prevention*** **and** ***control*** of communicable diseases and infection at local (i.e. District) level," as this precise accountability had never before been so clearly spelt out. It is worth exploring these concepts in greater detail.

The term "surveillance" has so many possible interpretations that it is important to have a clear understanding of its meaning in this context. Perhaps the briefest definition might be "obtaining information for action." A more comprehensive one would, of course, go into much greater detail. Many of the latter have been described by epidemiologists during the past 60 years or so, but that set out by Last (1983) is often quoted as being one of considerable usefulness and applicability: "The ongoing scrutiny of systematically collected data, generally using methods distinguished by their practicability, uniformity and frequently their rapidity rather than complete accuracy. Its main purpose is to detect changes in trends or distribution in order to initiate investigation and control measures." Noah (2006) has expressed the view that the only factor which he would add is that the information should be "timely for action." Curiously enough this concept of surveillance was not totally new in England. Mention was made in Chap. 3 of the amateur efforts of the wealthy haberdasher John Graunt in studying the patterns and distribution of deaths in London, along with their reported causes. However such an approach could only be seen as strategic, pointing out "black spots" for carefully considered attention. In as much as it referred to mortality it could hardly be said to meet Noah's criterion quoted above! But it was not until the late 1950s that a *national* surveillance system which was "timely for action" could be said to exist in England. This came about when Dr W Charles Cockburn of the PHLS developed a system by which all public health laboratories submitted weekly microbiological reports to a national centre at Colindale. This arrangement allowed him to produce a simple weekly picture of infection in England in the form of a brief report which could be circulated throughout the country to those who needed to know or who were professionally interested. Furthermore, as mentioned above, it was not until the Acheson Report of 1988 that *local, district, surveillance* became a formal requirement.

The media have, of course, familiarised us with the word as it is used e.g. in news items concerning the security services or in police television dramas, in which it refers to on-going vigilance concerning the activities of particular individuals, groups or organisations. In fact, until around 1950, in public health practice also it tended to refer to the monitoring of individuals who were contacts of cases of a serious communicable disease and who therefore required to be carefully observed for the possible development of early signs or symptoms. What changed from 1950 onwards was that Dr Alexander Langmuir, Chief of the Epidemiology Branch of CDC Atlanta, USA began to apply the term to specific diseases and to populations rather than to single individuals.

Much of the above illustrates very well the need to define clearly the use of the word surveillance in whatever situation one finds oneself. For example, in 1994, while participating in a post-doctoral seminar at a university department of epidemiology in the United States, I emphasised that it had not been until 1988 that setting up a fully developed surveillance system at district level had become mandatory in England. I had obviously expressed myself badly and my comment was considerably misunderstood. It soon became obvious that my American colleagues were using the term communicable disease *surveillance* to cover the entire range of public health activities from reporting through to control, and I quickly had to assure them that in England infectious diseases had not simply been allowed to run riot until 1988! I had, in fact, been using the term to convey the concept of a complete local surveillance system including clinical notifications, laboratory reports, analysis of data, monitoring of trends, feedback to those to need to know etc. and this did not become a formal District requirement until that year. I came across a similar opportunity for confusion when working as an external consultant to the European Commission in 2004. In the country which I was visiting I was assured that a well-developed surveillance system was in operation but I found that in practice this simply meant that there was a list of diseases which had to be notified to the public health authority. This is not to deny the fundamental importance of notification or reporting as before a public health authority can set in place any control measures it has, of course, to be aware of the incident. Chapter 3 described how notification of cases was introduced in England but earlier informal methods must have existed, however undependable. More recently laboratory reporting has become more significant, a facility witnessed rather earlier in the United States than in England, although now fully developed in the latter.

Having explored the origins of surveillance in some detail and emphasised its critical importance, one can now turn to control and prevention, but attention first needs to be drawn to the interrelationship between the latter two. An example of what might be regarded as *primary* prevention is protection by e.g. immunisation, i.e. in which the immune status of the individual personally is altered in a manner leading to protection against a specific disease. *Secondary* prevention could be conceived of as the beneficial effect to the individual of a source of infection having been dealt with or a path of transmission being interrupted; for example, *control* of infectious case A by isolation *prevents* the infection of susceptible individual B, and the use of a condom can help to reduce the risk of acquiring—or spreading—HIV or other sexually-transmitted infections. The entire concept of the interlinked processes of control/prevention can most readily be understood by focusing on the three key elements of, logically, *source of infection*, *path of transmission*, and *susceptible individual*. Examples of the three elements are given in Diagrams X, XX, and XXX.

Cases of infectious disease.

Contacts of such a case, who may be developing the disease.

Carriers of infectious disease.

Domestic or pet animals, which may be sources of a variety of infections or infestations e.g. Toxocara from dogs or cats, Brucellosis, Pathogenic E.Coli, and Salmonellosis from cattle.

The physical environment itself, e.g. Tetanus from soil, Anthrax from soil or imported hides, Leptospirosis from pools infected by rat urine, Lyme Disease from infected ticks on vegetation, and Legionnaires' Disease from water in cooling towers.

(In warmer climates, of course, e.g. Malaria, Dengue Fever, and Yellow Fever from infected mosquitoes.)

Diagram X Sources of infection

Action taken by individual:

Covering the mouth in coughing and the nose in sneezing

Hand-washing before eating

Hygienic food-handling

Use of protective clothing/facemasks when appropriate

Hygienic handling of livestock, domestic pets etc.

Use of condoms

Avoiding injecting drug misuse

Avoiding swimming in quarries, open pools, or other infected waters

Avoiding exposure to deer ticks on bracken, shrubbery etc.

(Use of mosquito nets in warmer climates)

Action taken by various authorities:

Isolation of cases or carriers of infectious disease; quarantine of contacts

Cleaning, disinfection, sterilisation etc. of premises and materials

Exclusion of infectious individuals from e.g. work or school

Ensuring safety in importation, storage and preparation of food

Pasteurisation of milk

Purification of public water supplies

Sterilisation of imported hides etc.

Chemical treatment of water in cooling towers

Screening of blood etc. for donation

Diagram XX Cutting across paths of transmission

It would be tempting—and perhaps predictable—at this stage to describe progress in this field under three headings such as: which infectious diseases have been conquered, which are currently being tackled, and which we may have to face in the future. There are two reasons for my not adopting this approach, namely that this material (especially the first of these) has already been widely written about elsewhere, and also it would in my view "de-personalise" a chapter which I would prefer to treat in an individualistic manner. And so instead, what I have done is to select one example relating to each category which gives an indication of my

Vaccination/Immunisation against:

Smallpox

***Diphtheria**

***Whooping-cough**

***Tetanus**

Tuberculosis

***Poliomyelitis**

***Measles**

***Mumps**

***Rubella**

Haemophilus Influenzae **type b (Hib)**

Influenza

***Meningococcal infection**

***Pneumococcal infection**

***Human papillomavirus infection**

***Routinely offered as part of the Health Protection Agency's Childhood Immunisation Schedule. (Protection against Anthrax, Cholera, Hepatitis A, Hepatitis B, Rabies, Typhoid Fever, Chickenpox, and Yellow Fever is available in England only for specific clinical, occupational or travel reasons.)**

Diagram XXX Protection of susceptible individual

personal view of its importance vis-à-vis the others, namely, childhood immunisation, tuberculosis, and pandemic influenza.

Routine childhood immunisation is aimed at reducing morbidity and mortality from vaccine-preventable diseases. In the Developing World it stands alongside clean drinking water as a major determinant of individual, family and community health because of its contribution to the control and ultimate eradication of specific infectious diseases. More than two million children die needlessly each year because they have not received appropriate immunisations. It is equally important in the Developed World. Additionally, there is ample evidence that a very large number of immunising agents can *safely* be given simultaneously without loss of the individual constituents (Offit 2011).

I must personally confess to holding the view that immunisation represents one of the most successful achievements in preventive medicine. When one talks of preventing e.g. coronary heart disease, one is really reflecting simply *reducing the risk* by screening and by modifying lifestyle factors such as smoking, diet and exercise, along with treatment for hypertension or raised blood cholesterol etc. When one refers to preventing poliomyelitis, however, the outcome is (almost) absolute rather than relative—immunisation gives (near) total protection from the disease. My convictions have been strengthened by the fact that from 1976 to 1990 I was fortunate enough to be co-opted to represent the NHS on the Medical Research Council's Committee for the Development of Vaccines and Immunisation Procedures—essentially to act as a modest part of the interface between laboratory science and service provision, as it were. Although my prime role in being there was to consider the practicability and acceptability of offering new or modified vaccines within the health service, I was inevitable that I was uniquely exposed not only to a profound understanding of the value of these preventive measures but also to the Council's ethical approach to all vaccine trials, from reactogenicity (what were the reactions to the vaccine being given?), immunogenicity (did appropriate levels of e.g. antibodies develop?), and effectiveness (was disease prevented?) It was significant that only volunteers from the Council's own staff took part in the first of these.

Our immune system, which has an evolutionary history of around 400 million years (Ogunmekan 1996), has developed (and also, of course, has been further helped on its way by immunisation) to provide a measure of protection against infectious agents. Immunity is generally classified as *innate* or *acquired.*

Innate immunity derives principally from the genetic constitution of the individual, providing non-specific cellular responses by phagocytes which can help to destroy microorganisms. A group of plasma proteins called "complement" increase the protective effect of these cells.

Acquired immunity can be achieved naturally by encountering a particular pathogen (and, of course, surviving the infection!) or artificially by the process of *active* or *passive* immunisation.

Active immunisation is carried out using antigens, i.e. inactivated or killed vaccines (e.g. pertussis), live vaccines (e.g. BCG), or toxoids (e.g. diphtheria), according to the disease against which protection is sought. The protective responses are therefore highly specific for a particular microorganism and consist of the release of antibodies from B-lymphocytes and the production of T-lymphocytes which can help phagocytes to destroy the invading pathogen. The first immunisation procedure may not result in an adequate level of antibody production. A second procedure, carried out after an appropriate interval, may however create an antibody response which is not only considerably greater but also much longer-lasting. Further procedures may be necessary to achieve and maintain protection against any particular infection.

Passive immunisation is achieved by injecting immunoglobulins derived from the blood of human donors, thereby conferring immediate though temporary protection against specific diseases. The immunoglobulins used may be derived from pooled plasma of blood donors and are therefore able to offer a measure of protection against infections which are common or against which immunisation is a routine procedure in the local population. There are also specific immunoglobulins derived from persons who have recently experienced the specific disease or immunised against it. Lastly "natural" passive immunity occurs when antibodies, from either previous maternal infection or immunisation, are transferred to the baby via the placenta and also in the colostrum of early feeding.

What is referred to as **herd immunity** is simply the immunity of a group, representing the resistance to the spread of infection within that group based on the proportion of its individual members who are immune by virtue of either natural acquisition or having been immunised. If that proportion is sufficiently large, it may provide indirect protection to some non-immunised children, who are shielded from infection by a "protective wall" of immunised individuals. Differing perceptions of the value of herd immunity raise some important practical and ethical questions. On the one hand, this property is understandably attractive to those responsible for organising public health programmes; on the other hand, parents are primarily concerned with the health, welfare and safety of their *own* children. In the Developed World particularly, these differences in perception can have a profound effect on not only to what extent people trust their government on these issues but also the extent to which they regard their general medical practitioners as "instruments" of government policy. The implications for public education programmes are clear, especially in countries like England where the arrangements are entirely voluntary (unlike e.g. France, the United States, or Malta, where at least some of the procedures are, directly or indirectly, required by law).

The introduction of "artificial" immunity by the use of antigens has quite a long history. Variolation—the attempt to produce immunity against smallpox by inoculating a person with pus taken from an active lesion of someone suffering from the disease—was practised in the East as far back as the sixteenth century. The story is well known of Lady Wortley Montague, wife of the British ambassador in Constantinople, arranging for her own children to receive this, and on her return home in 1721 successfully promoting the procedure in England. Not unexpectedly 1–3% died of smallpox induced by the variolation (Parish 1965) and in 1768 a number of cases of secondary encephalomyelitis were described by Dr Rechberger of Vienna (Wilson 1967). In spite of these fatalities, the popularity of variolation clearly meant that the public had felt that the risk was worth taking, given that at the time the disease had a mortality rate of up to 20% (Link 2005), an early indication that the concept of risk/benefit analysis had become publicly understood to some extent.

The literature of the origins of smallpox vaccination and its introduction in England following Dr Jenner's successful vaccination of the 8-year old James Phipps in 1796 is voluminous, but the following brief account is sufficient for the present purpose. On 14th May 1796 Jenner used lymph from a cowpox pustule on the wrist of a milkmaid to inoculate the boy. The outcome is perhaps best by Jenner's own comment:

> *On the first of July following, this boy was inoculated with matter immediately taken from a smallpox pustule.............but no disease followed.*

Jenner published his findings in 1798 *An Inquiry into the causes and effects of the variolae vaccinae, a disease discovered in some of the Western counties of England particularly Gloucestershire and known by the name of cowpox.* It is, of course, quite well known that Jenner was not the first person in England to carry out an experiment along these lines. In 1774 a Dorset cattle breeder named Benjamin Jesty had used matter from "pap-pox" to inoculate his wife and two young children. Although this procedure appeared to protect them against smallpox, his wife's arm became so inflamed that she had to be treated by a surgeon (Creighton 1894).

What are perhaps more important however in a historical sense, are both the professional and public reactions to the Government's subsequent adoption of smallpox vaccination in what might be regarded as a crusading spirit, prompted by epidemics of the disease. Doctors varied in their reaction its introduction but Dr John Sims of London in a letter to a medical journal in 1799, made the point that doctors should be careful to avoid accusations of introducing the new disease of cowpox, given that they were unable to cure many existing diseases. A further reservation was expressed on behalf of those who believed that vaccination was "sinful and doubting of Providence;" in fact, the concept of interfering with God's Providence persisted for many years as one of the most effective arguments against vaccination (Stern 1927). Lastly some of the alternative (traditional) practitioners of the day were none too pleased at this addition to the physician's scientific armamentarium as it threatened to undermine their earnings (Durbach 2005). However the effectiveness of vaccination in reducing mortality from smallpox was proved by 1800, deaths falling slowly but steadily from 7,347 in 1798 to 6,560 in 1802, and 4,667 in 1806. And by 1837 doctors were able to show that unvaccinated persons were much more at risk (Smith 1979).

In England, as Porter (1997) has described, Victorian society had many advocates of state medicine whose ideology included the belief that the sovereign right of the individual to contract and spread infection should be regarded as less important than the right of the whole community to be protected, a sort of epidemiological aspect of utilitarianism. It was against this background that the Vaccination Act of 1840 made the procedure available to all by the appointment of Public Vaccinators, and an amendment in the following year declared that it was to be at public cost. In spite of this, there was considerable public reluctance to take advantage of this. The Government's determination resulted in its passing the Vaccination Act of 1853, which made the procedure compulsory for infants before the age of 4 months. Perhaps not surprisingly, within a few months the Anti-Vaccination League was founded and because of counter-propaganda and heated controversy this Act was very rarely enforced.

However in 1871 smallpox again began to represent a serious problem and Hardy (1993) has commented that that year represented a watershed in the history of smallpox in London because it saw the establishment of "the stamping-out policy" against the disease. Further legislation made it clear that compulsion was to be taken seriously, with prosecutions for those parents who refused. Bitter public opposition now ensued, leading to considerable social disturbance, public demonstrations and riots, especially over the issue of the threat of sending parents to jail for this offence. Welshman (2000) describes how the city of Leicester had, by 1885, become known as the centre of the anti-compulsory vaccination movement, having been the scene of the most violent riots,; additionally the City's vaccination rate for children dropped from 90% in 1872 to just 3% by 1892.

As Stern (1927) has recounted, in 1885, by which time thousands of parents had been summoned and a few jailed, widespread public demonstrations showed that opposition to compulsion was so vehement that the law could no longer operate. In the closing years of the century, the concept of "conscientious objection" was introduced following the report of a Royal Commission, even though the infant's father required to go to Court to affirm this. By 1907, it had become sufficient for the father to provide a sworn declaration before a Justice of the Peace. In the same year, by a curious coincidence, the first recorded case of post-vaccinal encephalitis was described by a French physician (Comby 1907). Subsequent cases were noted in England, the first being a patient in the London Hospital in 1912 (Turnbull and McIntosh 1926). To this has to be added the contribution of some of the more grotesque examples of simple folklore: there were widespread fears that children exposed to this "bestial procedure" would develop horns and undergo transformation of their human character (Dudgeon 1963). Accordingly the reservations which many members of the public felt about the procedure were not simply based on the infringement of their civil liberties.

As was mentioned in Chap. 4 (in connection with diphtheria inoculation), theoretically the law on compulsion was not finally withdrawn until 1946, with the passing of the National Health Service Act, which made no mention of any legal requirement, but in practice the unpopularity of any kind of compulsion meant that the law had continued to play a diminishing role. For example, neither my father nor I received smallpox vaccination as infants, a situation which we both had cause to regret when we subsequently had to have the procedure carried out as adults—a much more unpleasant experience—during an actual smallpox outbreak.

Fortunately such outbreaks are now a thing of the past. In spite of the earlier problems of its acceptance, vaccination was finally the means by which the disease was eradicated worldwide. A WHO global eradication project which began modestly in 1959, as a result of an initiative from the Soviet Union, eventually achieved fulfilment in October 1977 when the last naturally acquired case was tracked down in Somalia as a result of a relentless campaign of surveillance, control and prevention. The individual who bore this distinction was a hospital cook and it is gratifying to be able to record that he recovered from the infection. In spite of this monumental success, representing a phenomenal degree of international cooperation over a couple of decades, it was not until December 1979 that the Global Commission for the Eradication of Smallpox felt able to declare the world free of the disease, following which routine vaccination ceased to be offered. On a slightly more selfish note, a particular nightmare had been removed from the lives of public health doctors like myself! [Smallpox virus samples continue to exist in secure conditions in two laboratories, one in the United States and the other in Russia. Whilst some anxieties are expressed about the risks implicit in this situation, a number of researchers have pleaded for these samples not to be destroyed as they may be required to create vaccines against any related virus such as monkey pox.]

Diphtheria immunisation, the first protective procedure to be offered to children after smallpox vaccination, was dealt with in Chap. 4, the only point worth making once more being the regret that its introduction in England was greatly delayed, which Mortimer (2010, Personal communication. Letter to author 19th February 2010) described as "an opportunity missed throughout the 1930s." I have an embarrassing memory of an event which occurred while carrying out a diphtheria immunisation session quite early in my professional life. In the late 1950s one had to carry out a preliminary Schick test—intradermal injection of 0.1 ml Diphtheria Toxin—and view the result 1 week later. If the test was positive, i.e. the injected area showed inflammation, then the child was susceptible to the disease and the protective injection could be given. If not, no injection was given as it was considered that the child had acquired immunity from subclinical infection, which was still quite common in those days, and it was best to avoid an unacceptable reaction. (The toxoids available at that time were not as purified as present day antigens.) Both toxin and toxoid were produced by the same manufacturer and, unfortunately from one point of view, came in the same size of bottle and had a similar-coloured label. In a very busy clinic session I unwittingly gave a child a dose of the toxin in the belief that it was the protective antigen. I always kept the two materials at opposite ends of the table but on this occasion someone had moved them and I did not double check before giving the injection—a mistake I was careful *never* to repeat. As soon as I realised what I had done I informed the child's mother and, with the help of a nurse, kept the child under observation at home for 48 h. The child remained perfectly well, fortunately, and I had been somewhat reassured when my head of department (whom I had telephoned immediately) told me that he had once done the same thing!

Pertussis immunisation using a vaccine made from whole, killed *Bordetella Pertussis* cells was, in the late 1950s, next to be introduced into the routine immunisation schedule, from 1961 being combined with diphtheria and tetanus to form the so-called triple vaccine (DPT). The impact on the occurrence of the disease was early and dramatic. In 1972, when vaccine acceptance was over 80%, the incidence had been cut to just 2% of the pre-immunisation levels. By 1975, however, public concern over the safety of the vaccine because of reports of possible brain damage had reduced acceptance to just 30% and the incidence of the disease reverted to its previous levels of around 100,000 (Salisbury et al. 2006). In fact, the early development of the vaccine had never been quite trouble-free.; as far back as 1933 Madsen had reported a fatal case of encephalopathy following administration of the vaccine. Parental anxieties over this matter were readily understandable. Sometimes febrile reactions to the pertussis component could be quite frightening. I gave my own daughter her first DPT injection at age 3 months and, to our horror, she was extremely ill as a result, becoming limp, pale and unresponsive. I did not continue with the remainder of the DPT course but there was a penalty to this. When she was 3 years old she developed the disease and my wife and I had probably the most worrying 3 or 4 days of our lives, standing by her waiting—interminably, it seemed—for her to breathe again after each prolonged paroxysm of coughing. I never again doubted the word of other parents who had horrific stories to tell. (Vaccination against poliomyelitis was also introduced in the 1950s, initially as a killed vaccine in 1956 offered via mass campaigns aimed at all those under 40 years of age, but subsequently as a live vaccine in 1962 for incorporation into the routine childhood immunisation schedule. I covered this issue in Chap. 5 as it was relevant to my duties as a public health doctor in Stockport at the time.)

Nevertheless, in as much as genuine medical contraindications to immunisation are extremely rare, it becomes relevant to ask why it is not the case that virtually all children are given this valuable protection. Apart from countries in which some at least of the procedures are obligatory, the attitudes of parents are clearly of paramount importance. In England it used to be commonly said that those who did not present their children for immunisation were "feckless" or in some other way lacking in a sense of responsibility. However a piece of research carried out in Coventry in 1984 by Middleton and Pollock showed that immunisation consent forms had been completed by over 90% of parents but that many general practitioners (and, on their behalf, their practice receptionists) were excluding children because of supposed, but irrelevant, contraindications, resulting in a take-up of only 42%. The Peckham Report (1989) revealed similar hurdles in that general practitioners' misconceptions, at that time, about contraindications to measles and pertussis immunisation had had a major influence, confirmed by the explanations given by parents for their child not being immunised.

Parents' attitudes and behaviour can sometimes be adversely influenced by a wide range of factors: they may take the view that "these dangerous germs no longer exist in England—we never hear of a case of diphtheria these days;" or conversely they may worry about a number of a number of different antigens being given simultaneously ("overloading" the immune system, although there is ample evidence that this is certainly *not* the case); lack of convenient local clinic or even transport facilities may present practical problems; some mothers with several children and no support may simply find it impossible to attend immunisation session; the views of grandparents and other (usually older) relations may affect judgment; cultural and religious beliefs may play a part even in the Developed World; the effects of the media can be quite profound, especially when they appear to emphasis risk rather than present the case in an even-handed manner; (this last point is brought out particularly in what might be described as the "MMR saga" below).

It may be useful to pause at this point and give some general thoughts to the media in the general sphere of health. It may be tempting to believe that they should be in some kind of positive partnership with health care professionals as far as medical issues are concerned. However Watts (2006), a freelance science and medical writer and broadcaster, wrote recently "*Journalism is not about health education... it is about stories that interest people. Nor do reporters and broadcasters owe their first loyalty to the health care community. Their loyalty is to their readers, listeners and viewers, who will go elsewhere if they are unsatisfied.*" He pointed out that, additionally, journalists may not have the last word on what is actually published as sub-editors and editors may wish to give the material their own particular "slant." The outcome of this is that a health professional, for example, may feel that information given to a journalist has not been presented in the correct light. Local media may have a rather different approach as key individuals have the opportunity to get to know one another and may be able to achieve a mutually beneficial working relationship. For example, I spent 27 years as the public health spokesman for infectious disease matters in Coventry which meant that I had had the opportunity to get to know—in some cases very well—the editors and health correspondents of the *Coventry Evening Telegraph* along with the producers of both the local radio station and regional television. In the case of the local press, for instance, a common arrangement would be for me to discuss a health issue (such as an outbreak of typhoid) with the newspaper's health correspondent, I being accountable for the factual information and the journalist deciding on the appropriate slant of the proposed news item or feature. An element of trust was involved as each had to be fully understanding of the other's role and responsibilities. With regard to the national media, such collaboration must be difficult for a locally-based health professional to achieve and so it is in this sector that the problems seem to arise.

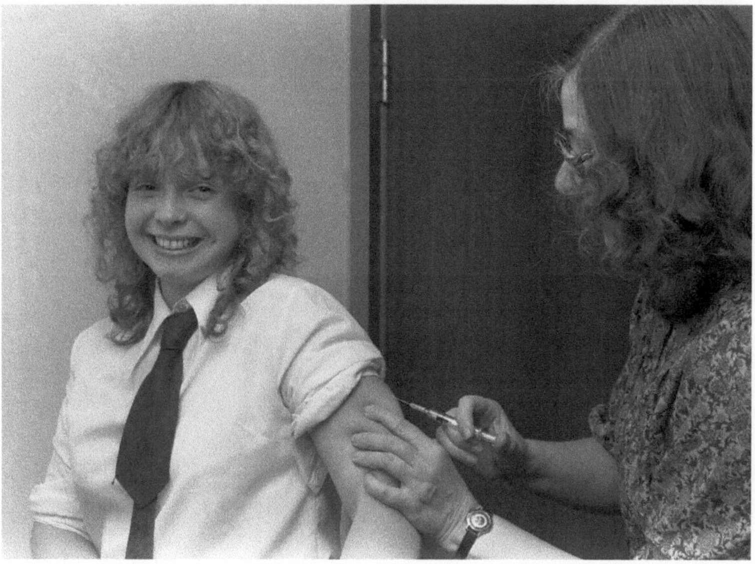

When the measles vaccine was introduced into the immunisation schedule in 1968, take-up was never high enough to cut across measles virus transmission and by the late 1980s annual notifications had fallen only to between 50,000 and 100,000. Nevertheless this compared favourably with the pre-immunisation situation when notifications ranged from 160,000 to 800,000 depending on whether the year was a "measles" or "non-measles" one (Salisbury et al. 2006). In as much as countries with high take-up of the vaccine (such as the United States, where the procedure was required as a condition of school entry) had shown that a major impact could be made on the incidence of the disease, it was important to try to find ways of encouraging parents to take advantage of the facility. Some of my young colleagues in the Department of Community Medicine in Coventry, in conjunction with the creative director of an advertising agency, had the ingenious idea of adopting an off-beat, non-traditional approach by running a poster campaign in 1985 with the message:

Question: *What can you get in Coventry that you can't get in New York, San Francisco or Los Angeles?*

Answer: Measles!

(The idea was that the small print of the answer would make it likely that people would take the trouble to look carefully to see it, and therefore would find it surprising and, we hoped, thought-provoking.)

Vaccination against rubella was introduced in stages, initially in 1970 for pre-pubertal girls and non-immune women of child-bearing age in order to prevent rubella infection in pregnancy and the "congenital rubella syndrome." In 1977 a concentrated campaign focused on girls in the 11–14 age bracket and 2 years later a national campaign was launched specifically aimed at women of child-bearing age. The illustration shows my 15-year old daughter putting on a brave smile as she receives the injection. It was, of course, imperative to avoid accidentally vaccinating someone who might be pregnant and I am glad to say that the question "Do you have any reason to believe you might be pregnant?" did not seem to cause offence (although it did result in a certain amount of good-natured amusement at girls' schools!)

It was not until 1988, when the combined measles/mumps/rubella (MMR) vaccine was introduced that more satisfactory coverage against measles was achieved, because of its obvious appeal to parents, one combined antigen protecting against three diseases and only two injections instead of six. Levels of protection rose to over 90% and it would have indeed been difficult to foresee the situation which was to develop in 1998.

The problem arose when the *Lancet*, a medical journal with a high international reputation, published in February 1998 a paper by a group of researchers at the Royal Free Hospital in London (Wakefield et al. 1998) which suggested a link between the MMR vaccine and the development of autism, thereby launching a health scare of a nature and extent almost certainly never previously experienced. There were very soon many scientific criticisms of both the research itself and the decision of the *Lancet* to publish it; for example, the research involved only 12 children who moreover did not appear to have represented a random sample. Over the following decade an overwhelming amount of scientifically validated research subsequently showed that there was no epidemiological evidence for a causal association between the vaccine and autism. Additionally in February 2004 ten of Dr Wakefield's co-signatories issued a "partial retraction" of the 1998 paper. However, to quote Dr Richard Horton, the *Lancet's* Editor, Dr Wakefield and his colleagues "had lit the fuse of a gunpowder trail that could not be extinguished" (Horton 2004).

By the time the paper was finally retracted 12 years later, not only had it been shown that it was fatally flawed both scientifically and ethically, but was also an elaborate fraud (Godlee et al. 2011). Consequently Dr Wakefield and his senior co-author Dr John Walker-Smith were struck off the UK Medical Register, after the General Medical Council's longest ever fitness to practise hearing. Unfortunately the damage to confidence in the immunisation procedure had been done. It was predicted that this would precipitate a vaccine scare, with reduced vaccine uptake and a return of measles outbreaks, and this turned out to have been a correct forecast (Bedford and Elliman 2010). A "ripple effect" was also noted in that the anxiety which had been created led to a slightly diminished take-up of *all* vaccines in the immunisation programme. Fortunately MMR vaccination rates in England are now rising: the NHS Information Centre figures show that in 2009/2010 88.2% of children had had the procedure carried out, and by the following year the Health Protection Agency was able to show that the figure had reached 90% for the first time in 13 years. However this is still significantly short of the World Health Organisation's target for optimum herd immunity which is 95%.

Mention has been made above of the important role which the media can play with regard to health issues generally. Certainly their handling of the MMR scare shows just how much damage can be done to a disease-prevention programme by giving equal coverage to an individual piece of discredited research alongside the opposing conclusions of the wealth of scientific research of the highest professional standing, and continuing to do so even years after the matter had been settled, giving the impression that they are reluctant to leave the matter behind and move on. For example an article in the *Daily Mail* on 31 October 2005 was headed "**MMR safe? Baloney. This is one scandal that's getting worse**," this being the newspaper's response to the recent publication of a Cochrane systematic review (surely the most rigorous test of any research topic) concluding that there was no credible evidence of a link between MMR and autism. Television has also been guilty of continuing to promote the idea that there may yet be some doubt concerning the safety of the vaccine. As recently as 10 February 2006, the extremely popular BBC courtroom soap *Judge John Deed* had a story based on a mother refusing to let her baby have the MMR vaccine because of her conviction that it was dangerous.

The impact of words, especially in headlines, is something that journalists understand very well. Public health spokespersons fortunate enough to receive training in dealing with the media are likely to have some of this wisdom passed on to them. They may find the guidance counter-intuitive: instead of the characteristic scientific paper–type approach (i.e. Introduction/Background, Methodology, Results, and Conclusions etc., gradually working up to the "impact point") they may be exhorted to state the findings *first*—in bold headlines—and provide the supporting information beneath the banner, almost as reference material.

What may require closer study, however, is the capacity for the particular wording of an item unwittingly to convey an incorrect—and anxiety-provoking—impression. For example the Channel 4 News item on 21st February 2004 headed "*New MMR Controversy*" was not, as might have been imagined, based on some new evidence casting doubt on the safety of the vaccine. Far from it—-it was instead an account of the Health Secretary's call for an independent inquiry into the allegation that Dr Wakefield had failed to mention that he had been working on a study to see if there was evidence to support a legal action by parents claiming that the MMR vaccine had damaged their children. (On hearing that there had been this clear conflict of interest, the *Lancet* stated that, had they known this, they would not have published Dr Wakefield's paper in the first instance.) As a further example of this phenomenon,

Brian Deer's television documentary "*MMR: What the doctor didn't tell you*" was not a contribution to any conspiracy theory, but rather an indication that Dr Wakefield would shortly be due to answer charges of professional misconduct before the General Medical Council!

Introduced in 1992 (and perhaps almost forgotten as a result of the media "noise" over MMR) the Hib conjugate vaccine made a profound impact on the incidence of the serious invasive disease of young children, *haemophilus influenzae meningitis*, most markedly in the 2 year period after introduction: in children under 5 years of age, 803 cases in 1991, 80 in 1994, and only 21 in 1998. A similar success story can be relayed following the introduction in November 1999 of the *Meningococcal C* conjugate vaccine for children and young people up to the age of 18 years, extended in January 2002 up to 25 years of age. Cases fell by over 90% in all age groups immunised (Salisbury et al. 2006). A further protective measure was introduced in September 2006 by offering a *Pneumococcal* conjugate vaccine within the routine schedule. This vaccine resulted in immediate protection against seven of the forms of bacterial pneumococcal infection but was replaced in December 2009 by one which extended the protection against 13 forms. [Although the Human Papilloma Virus Vaccine was introduced in 2008 it is not proposed to include an account of this extremely valuable protective measure as the condition which it is intended to prevent—cervical cancer—is not an "infectious disease" in the sense in which the term is used in this book.]

As has been mentioned above, there has been no formal requirement for immunisation of children in England since the passing of the 1946 NHS Act. In fact, the concept of any kind of compulsion in this sphere had for many years before that been repugnant to the general public and, in fact, as far back as 1866 had been quietly and informally rejected by politicians as "doubtful whether it could be carried through Parliament" (Stern 1927). The fact that this latter issue related to smallpox vaccination is largely irrelevant; the general climate of opinion had been created. But there is a further factor which needs to be recognised in this respect. England has a tradition of being a secular, liberal democracy, reluctant to use the law in matters of personal health and generally content to rely on education and reasoned exhortation, supported by well organised provision of facilities.

How then, has this totally informal and voluntary English approach worked in practice? With the exception of the MMR vaccine (discussed above), the brief answer must be "surprisingly well." A number of factors contribute to this situation. Firstly, immunisation under the NHS is free and therefore there is no financial barrier to any child receiving the entire programme. Secondly, health promotion and information-giving begin early, beginning with the midwife during pregnancy and continuing with the health visitor when she takes over from the midwife when the infant is about 10 days old. Thirdly, a computerised system guarantees that entering the infant's data and parental consent into a child health database ensures that appropriate appointments are scheduled and details of immunisations given are recorded. Lastly, the fact that a significant proportion of general practitioners' remuneration depends on their achieving appropriate targets for immunisation coverage with regard to the children on their practice lists no doubt acts as a strong incentive to secure this objective.

At the end of Chap. 4 I stated that, from the perspective of the 1950s, it would have been difficult to believe that tuberculosis would not have been virtually eradicated from the country within a couple of decades or so, such had been the dramatic decline in its incidence due to a combination of improvements in living standards and the development of a succession of highly effective antibiotics, along with BCG vaccination. However, what might have been difficult to foresee was the great increase in immigration from countries with a high prevalence of the disease (especially sub-Saharan Africa, India, Pakistan and Bangladesh) along with the spread of HIV infection and the emergence of multi-drug resistance which rendered many standard treatment regimens ineffective (Donaldson and Scally 2009).

The significant increase in immigration, mainly from the countries of the Indian Sub-continent, had begun in the late 1950s but it was not until 1965 that what were referred to as Medical Arrangements for Long-stay Immigrants were introduced. In January of that year the Ministry of Health wrote to Medical Officers of Health stressing the importance of all such immigrants being visited so that they could be given general information about the National Health Service and persuaded to arrange to become registered with a general practitioner "with a view particularly to having a chest X-ray where appropriate" (Ministry of Health 1965a). This emphasis on the chest X-ray was explained in the letter which the Ministry sent to all general practitioners pointing out the importance of "securing by voluntary action that those from countries with a high incidence of tuberculosis—particularly from Asia—should have a chest X-ray as soon as possible after their arrival in the country" (Ministry of Health 1965b).

There was, in fact, an initial post-war decline in the disease, a plateau from 1985 to 1991, and a subsequent increase. To the extent to which this increase was due to immigration it was felt that three factors could be operating. For example, In the 1970 Annual Report of the Medical Officer of Health of Coventry (Clayton 1970), a city with a significant proportion of persons from India (mainly Punjab) and Pakistan, the following entry appeared: "*Because of the relatively long incubation period of tuberculosis, it is rarely easy to state whether the patient 1. became infected after his arrival in this country (possibly because of living in overcrowded conditions), 2. was incubating the condition on arrival, or 3. was suffering from tuberculosis prior to leaving his/her country of origin. Only when a routine chest X-ray is required of all intending immigrants in their country of origin will this problem be controlled. The recent developments for X-ray examination at the main airports in the United Kingdom have gone some way towards meeting the problem and gratitude must be expressed to the Health Control staff at these airports who so promptly notify local Health Departments of those immigrants who appear to require investigation for tuberculosis.*"

In Coventry, as in other parts of England with a relatively high immigrant population, the situation reflected continuing cause for concern and it was considered that measures for the prevention and control of the disease in the city should be intensified. In 1971, and again in 1988, additional efforts were directed towards these objectives by promptly recognising and treating cases along with screening and active case-finding amongst family and other close contacts. An important factor was ensuring that patients did in fact comply with their treatment and complete the course. In my 1989 Report as Director of Public Health of Coventry Health Authority (Pollock 1989) I laid heavy emphasis on the fact that although only 62 cases of tuberculosis had been notified during the year the death rate in Coventry from this disease was the highest in the country. Although I retired from this post in 1990 I was pleased to note that my successor, Dr Keith Williams, vigorously continued these efforts and his first Annual Report shows what a high degree of priority he and his colleagues had allocated to this on-going problem. In spite of this, new notifications of tuberculosis in Coventry were at the same level in 1999 as in 1988.

More recently in England, as Pareek et al. (2011) have shown, National guidance for screening has been hampered by lack of data concerning the prevalence of latent tuberculosis in immigrants. Based on their multicentre cohort study, they recommend screening of individuals from countries with an incidence of the disease of more than 250 cases per 100,000, or more than 150 cases per 100,000 (if immigrants from the Indian subcontinent are included) as they have shown that this should detect 92% of infected immigrants. Additional emphasis on the need for some such approach has been provided by Abubakar et al. (2011) who have drawn attention to the fact that, because of immigration, the disease is increasing in England at a time when it is declining in most parts of Western Europe. They have declared that it is time to regain control of this situation, also drawing attention to the deficiencies of the current screening programme, but in addition outlining urgent control measures including prompt detection in such groups as homeless people and asylum seekers, and more effective treatment regimes. The particular vulnerability of HIV-affected persons to tuberculosis has been known for some considerable time and is best dealt with by close consultation between the various specialists who may be involved. Similarly, multi-drug-resistant tuberculosis will continue to require ingenuity in the development and use of antibiotics.

Perhaps the greatest anxiety with regard to the future is the threat that Influenza AH5N1 (or another influenza virus) will mutate and cause a true pandemic with very high mortality. The particular fear concerning AH5N1 is that it is now widespread globally in the bird population and, although up till now humans have only become infected directly from bird sources, it might take only a minor mutation to result in human to human transmission (Ladhani 2010). In Chap. 7 reference was made to the Chief Medical Officer's warning in 2005 regarding the effects of an influenza pandemic—the enormous pressure on health care facilities and the targeting of those services at those most in need. It has now become obvious that many people believe that "bringing the big guns to bear" on the 2009/2010 AH1N1 pandemic was a considerable over-reaction, and it may be that the danger now is that the public response to a pandemic caused by AH5N1 might be half-hearted (at least initially).

It is at least partially reassuring to be aware that, as soon as a new variant of the virus is identified and its pandemic potential realised, the intention is that steps be taken by vaccine manufacturers, working with the World Health Organisation's network of influenza reference laboratories, and with regulatory and standardisation authorities, to develop a pandemic specific vaccine and to attempt to manufacture enough to meet global needs. (Watson and Pebody 2011). These authors, however, point out that delay between virus recognition and production of a safe vaccine is a problem not yet solved and that what is needed are vaccines which protect against all forms of influenza. In the meantime, researchers from the US National Institutes of Health Vaccine Research Center have encouraged governments to launch vaccination programmes now to prevent a AH2N2 pandemic, as immunity against this strain is very low in people aged under 50 and they believe that the strain could easily jump from animals and birds to humans (Nabel et al. 2011).

In the light of all the above it is to be hoped that, whatever the new structure emerging from the impending organisational changes may be, the CCDC will continue to operate within a supportive framework which must include the important element of "surge capacity." This element is best described as the ability to respond to whatever extent an acute situation demands. It depends on a prior understanding between a group of staff, both managers and their fieldworkers, that a particular situation will result in their being prepared to switch priorities for a limited time to provide all necessary support to the individual whose responsibility it is to handle the situation. The best example which I can personally recall was when, in 1968, there was an outbreak of cholera in a Spanish holiday resort and the Department of Health in London required all Medical Officers of Health to keep under surveillance for 5 days all persons returning from that resort. Notifications were received by telephone from a variety of airports and the requirement was that each person should be visited twice daily and have their temperature taken. In Coventry this amounted to twice daily surveillance of over 500 persons, and the only way in which I could possibly discharge this function was to call upon every district nurse, health visitor, midwife and public health inspector in the City to each take a small share of the 5-day load, with medical staff being reserved for rapid assessment of any doubtful case. No cases of cholera occurred in Coventry but it was gratifying to discover that staff could willingly and at short notice collaborate in this way. Another example of surge capacity was described in Chap. 7 in which, at the height of the AH1N1 pandemic, the scale of the response regarding both anti-virals and vaccination meant that large numbers of staff of the Sandwell Primary Health Care Trust and of the local authority had to be rapidly redeployed from their normal duties.

Let me end on an "off-beat" but, I hope, thought-provoking note. The first aeroplane that I ever flew in was not a holiday jet or a light aircraft; it was a Lancaster bomber (the Mark V version, known as the Lincoln). It was in 1955 when, as part of my National Service, I was Medical Officer to the 1st Battalion the King's Shropshire Light Infantry operating in the Aberdare Forest in Kenya during the Mau Mau uprising. During my leave I took advantage of the offer of a brief trip in this huge aircraft which, from its base at RAF Eastleigh, Nairobi, would be flying low over the bamboo forest trying to spot Mau Mau terrorist patrols. Surprisingly there was no spare space in the enormous machine where I might sit and the captain directed me to the only vacant position, the tail-gunner's turret, known as the "tailpiece." From there, in flight, I could of course only see where the plane had been, not where it was heading. And this book has, I suppose, reflected just such a viewpoint. In other words, this odyssey can only show how we have come to be where we are at the present time, and it is to be hoped that past misjudgements on the continuing risks from communicable diseases and the organisational arrangements required to prevent and control them will not be repeated.

References

Abubakar I et al (2011) Tuberculosis in the UK—time to regain control. BMJ 343:d4281

Adler MW (1987) The development of the venereal disease services. In: Farrow S (ed) The public health challenge. Hutchinson, London

Adler RE (2004) Medical firsts: from Hippocrates to the human genome. Wiley, Hoboken

Banks AL (1948) The development of the public health laboratory service in the eastern region. J R Soc Promot Health 68:229–236

Beaglehole R, Bonita R, Kjellstrom T (1993) Basic epidemiology. World Health Organisation, Geneva

Bede (731) Ecclesiastical history of the English people. Reprinted in 1975. Dent and Dutton, London/New York

Bedford HE, Elliman DA (2010) MMR vaccine and autism. BMJ 340:c655

Bentley FJ (1936) Artificial pneumothorax: experience of the London County Council. Medical research council special report series no. 215. HMSO, London

Bingham A (2005) The British popular press and venereal disease during the Second World War. Hist J 48:1055–1076. doi:10.1017/S0018246X05004917

Binysh JK, Chishty VA, Middleton JD, Pollock GT (1985) The health of Coventry. Coventry Health Authority, Coventry

Binysh JK, Chishty VA, Middleton JD, Pollock GT (1995) How to write—and use—the annual report of the director of public health. In: How to do it, vol 3. BMJ Publications, London

Bivins R (2007) 1961–1962 British smallpox outbreak. Immigr Minor 25(3):263–289

BMJ Editorial (1963) Lessons about smallpox. 10 August 1963

BMJ Editorial (1989) Control of hospital infection, 298. 28 January 1989

BMJ News Item (2010) 341:c5950. 30 October 2010

Booker J (2008) Maritime quarantine: the British experience c1650–1900. Ashgate Publishing Group, Farnham

Box K (1945) Diphtheria immunisation: an inquiry made by the social survey for the Ministry of Health. Ministry of Health, London

Brandt AM (1987) No magic bullet: a social history of venereal diseases in the United States. Oxford University Press 1985. Rev. Ed. 1987, Oxford

Buhier G (trans) (1886) The sacred books of the East, vol 25. Clarendon Press, Oxford

Butterworth E (1966) The 1962 smallpox outbreak and the British press. Race Class 7(4):347–364

Cartwright FF (1977) A social history of medicine. Longman, London/New York

Cartwright FF, Biddiss M (2000) Disease and history, 2nd edn. Sutton Publishing, Stroud

Chadwick E (1842) Report on an inquiry into the sanitary condition of the labouring population of Great Britain. Poor Law Commissioners, London

Chave SPW (1984) Oxford textbook of public health, vol 1. Oxford University Press, Oxford

G. Pollock, *An Epidemiological Odyssey: The Evolution of Communicable Disease Control*, DOI 10.1007/978-94-007-3998-7,

Churchill Sir WS (1956) History of the English-speaking peoples. Cassell, London
Cipolla CM (1976) Public health and the medical profession in the Renaissance. Cambridge University Press, Cambridge
City of Coventry Census (1831) Records. The Council House, Coventry
Clayton TM (1963) Annual report of the medical officer of health of Coventry for 1963. The Council House, Coventry
Clayton TM (1970) Annual report of the medical officer of health of Coventry for 1970. The Council House, Coventry
Cockburn A (1977) Where did our infectious diseases come from? The evolution of infectious disease. In: Elliott K, Whelan J (eds) Proceedings of CIBA foundation symposium, vol 49. Wiley, Chichester
Coker R (2006) Communicable disease control and contemporary themes in public health law. Public Health 120(Suppl. 1): 23–28
Comby J (1907) L'encéphalite aiguë chez les enfants. Archives de Médicine de l'Enfance 10:577
Creighton C (1894) A history of epidemics in Britain. Cambridge University Press, Cambridge
Cunliffe B (1983) The tribal islands. In: Crookston P (ed) The ages of Britain. Hamish Hamilton, London
Department of Health (1988) Public health in England: the report of the committee of inquiry into future development of the public health function. Chairman: Sir Donald Acheson. HMSO Cm 289, London
Department of Health (1989) Review of law on infectious disease control: consultation document. Department of Health, Stanmore
Department of Health (1990) Annual report of the chief medical officer: on the state of the public health. HMSO, London
Department of Health (1991) Annual report of the chief medical officer: on the state of the public health. HMSO, London
Department of Health (1995) Annual report of the chief medical officer: on the state of the public health. HMSO, London
Department of Health (1997) Annual report of the chief medical officer: on the state of the public health. HMSO, London
Department of Health (2005) Annual report of the chief medical officer: on the state of the public health. HMSO, London
Department of Health and Social Security (1970) The future structure of the national health service. HMSO, London
Department of Health and Social Security (1971) National health service reorganisation: consultative document. HMSO, London
Department of Health and Social Security (1972) Report of the working party on medical administrators, their function and training (the Hunter report). HMSO, London
Department of Health and Social Security (1973) Transitional arrangements and organisation and development of services: control of notifiable diseases and food poisoning. HRC(73)34, DHSS, London
Department of Health and Social Security (1974) Committee of enquiry report on the smallpox outbreak in London in March and April 1973 (the Cox report). HMSO, London
Department of Health and Social Security (1986a) The report of the committee of inquiry into an outbreak of food poisoning at Stanley Royd Hospital. HMSO Cmnd 9716, London
Department of Health and Social Security (1986b) First report of the committee of inquiry into the outbreak of Legionnaires' disease in Stafford in April 1985. HMSO Cmnd 9772, London
Department of Health and University of Surrey: Epidemiology and Public Health Research Unit (1989) Public health common data set. University of Surrey, Guildford
Department of Health/Public Health Laboratory Service (1995) Hospital infection control. (Second report of the committee chaired by Professor Mary Cooke.) HMSO, London
Dixon W (1832) Asiatic cholera at Sunderland. London Medical Gazette, 4 February 1832. Quoted in Creighton C (1894) A history of epidemics in Britain. Cambridge University Press, Cambridge

Donaldson LJ, Scally G (2009) Donaldson's essential public health, 3rd edn. Radcliffe Publishing, Oxford/New York

Douglas J, Edgar W (1962) Smallpox in Bradford, 1962. BMJ 1(5278):612–614

Dudgeon JA (1963) Development of smallpox vaccine in England in the eighteenth and nineteenth centuries. BMJ 1(5342):1367–1372

Durbach N (2005) Bodily matters: the anti-vaccination movement in England 1853–1907. Duke University Press, Durham

Earl D (1983) The Romans. In: Crookston P (ed) The ages of Britain. Hamish Hamilton, London

Edgeworth JA, Farmer M, Sicilia A et al (2011) Detection of prion infection in vCJD: a blood-based assay. Lancet 377:487–493

Faculty of Public Health *YouGov* Survey (2010) Faculty of public health, London

Farr W (1885) In: Humphreys NA (ed) Vital statistics: memorial volume of selections from the reports and writings of William Farr. Offices of the Sanitary Institute, London

Fenton MA (1882) Annual report of the medical officer of health of Coventry for 1882. Coventry History Centre, Coventry

Field S (2011) Public health England: the way ahead. Presentation at Birmingham City University, 17th May 2011

Fouchier RA, Kuiken T, Schutten M et al (2003) Aetiology: Koch's postulates fulfilled for SARS virus. Nature 423:240

Fracastoro G (1530) Syphilis sive Morbus Gallicus: a poem in Latin hexameters (trans: Wynne-Finch H (1935)). William Heinemann, London

Fracastoro G (1546) De Contagione et Contagiosis Morbis et Eorum Curatione. (Il Contagio le Malattie Contagiose e le loro Cura.) (Translation, introduction and notes by Prof. Vincenzo Busacchi (1950). Leo S Olschki, Florence

Fraser Brockington C (1965) Public health in the nineteenth century. E&S Livingston Ltd, Edinburgh/London

Fraser Brockington C (1966) A short history of public health. J&A Churchill Ltd, London

Frazer WM (1950) A history of English public health 1834–1939. Bailliere, Tindall and Cox, London

Galbraith NS (1967) A national epidemiological service. Public Health 81(5):221–228

Galbraith NS (1998) CDSC's origin and creation. Presentation at scientific programme marking 21st anniversary celebrations at CDSC, Colindale, 11 December 1998

Galbraith S (2002) Dr John Snow (1813–1858): his early years. Royal Institute of Public Health, London

General Board of Health (1854) Response to Dr John Snow's theory. General Board of Health, London

Godlee F, Smith J, Marcovitch H (2011) Wakefield's article linking MMR vaccine to autism was fraudulent. BMJ Editorial 342:c7452

Gooder A (1998) The black death in Coventry. Booklet no. 23, Coventry and County heritage series. Coventry Branch of the Historical Association, Coventry

Gostin LO (2000) Public health law: power, duty, restraint. University of California Press, Berkeley/Los Angeles/London

Gough JH, Barlow D, Holmes Sellors T, Thompson VC (1957) The results of thoracoplasty in the treatment of pulmonary tuberculosis. Thorax 12:241–252

Graunt J (1662) Natural and political observations upon the bills of mortality. Tho: Roycroft, for John Martin, James Allestry and Tho: Dicas, London

Hammonds EM (1993) The search for perfect control: a social history of diphtheria 1880–1930. PhD thesis. Harvard University, Boston

Hardy A (1993) The epidemic streets. Clarendon Press, Oxford

Harper DR (2004) Preparedness for SARS in the UK in 2003. Philos Trans R Soc Lond B 359:1131–1132

Hatcher J (2008) The black death: an intimate history. Weidenfeld and Nicolson, London

Health Protection Agency (2010a) About the HPA. HPA Website

Health Protection Agency (2010b) Epidemiological report of pandemic (H1N1) 2009 in the UK April 2009–May 2010. HPA Website
Hellerman C (2009) Swine flu not stoppable says WHO. CNN Health, 11 June 2009
Hermitage Day E (1924) The eve of the reformation. AR Mowbray & Co., London
Heymann DL, Rodier G (2004) Global surveillance, national surveillance, and SARS. Emerging infectious diseases. Medscape, 10 February 2004
Hickman T (2004) The call-up: a history of national service. Headline Book Publishing, London
Hippocrates (c400 BC) Of the Epidemics. Book 1. Translated by Francis Adams. The internet classics archive. http://classics.mit.edu/Hippocrates/epidemics.1.i.html
Holland WW, Stewart S (1997) Public health: the vision and the challenge. The Nuffield Trust, London
Horton R (2004) MMR: science and fiction. Granta Books, Cambridge
Howie Sir J (1970) Training of epidemiologists for control of communicable diseases. Proc R Soc Med (Section of epidemiology and preventive medicine) 63(5):519–521
Jefferson T, Del Mar C, Dooley L et al (2009) Physical interventions to interrupt or reduce the spread of respiratory viruses: systematic review. BMJ 339:b3675
John HH (1987) The medical officer of health. In: Farrow S (ed) The public health challenge. Hutchinson, London
Keevil JJ (1957) Medicine and the navy 1200–1900, vol 1. E&S Livingstone, Edinburgh/London
Kimberlin RH, Walker CA (1989) Pathogenesis of scrapie in mice after intragastric infection. Virus Res 12:213–220
Kinghorn HM (1921) Hermann Brehmer. Trans Am Clin Climatol Assoc 37:193–210
Ladhani S (2010) Childhood immunisation. Presentation at Birmingham Medical Institute 26 October 2010
Lambert R (1963) Sir John Simon 1816–1904. Macgibbon and Key, London
Landsborough Thomson A (1943) The organisation of a national public health laboratory service. Medical Research Council, London
Last JM (ed) (1983) A dictionary of epidemiology. Oxford University Press, New York
Lewis J (1991) The origins and development of public health in the UK. In: Holland WW, Detels R, Knox G (eds) Oxford textbook of public health, 2nd edn. Oxford University Press, Oxford
Link K (2005) The vaccine controversy: the history, use and safety of vaccination. Praeger, Westport
Longmate N (1966) King cholera. Hamish Hamilton, London
Macandrew R (1941) The red light: intimate hygiene for men and women of HM forces. Wales Publishing, London
Macnamara NC (1892) Asiatic cholera. Macmillan and Co., London
Madsen T (1933) Vaccination against whooping-cough. J Am Med Assoc 101:187
Major RA (1944) Agostino bassi and the parasitic theory of disease. Bull Hist Med 16:97–107
Massey A (1941) Annual report of the medical officer of Coventry for 1941. The Council House, Coventry
Maugham WS (1938) Sanatorium. I. The complete short stories of W Somerset Maugham II The world over (1952). Doubleday/Garden City, New York
McCrum R, MacNeil R, Cran W (1986) The story of English. Guild Publishing, Brighton
McGrew RE (1985) Encyclopedia of medical history. Macmillan Press, London
McKeown T (1979) The role of medicine. Basil Blackwell, Oxford
McNalty Sir AS (1953) The civilian health and medical services, vol 1. HMSO, London
Mead R (1720) A short discourse concerning pestilential contagion and the methods to be used to prevent it. Printed for Sam Buckley and Ralph Smith, London
Middleton JD, Pollock GT (1984) Measles immunisation levels. Lancet 1(8369):167–168 [Letter]
Midland Daily Telegraph 7th September 1937. Coventry History Centre Archives, Jordan Well, Coventry
Milne Sir D (1964) The Aberdeen typhoid outbreak 1964: report of the departmental committee of enquiry. HMSO, Edinburgh
Ministry of Health (1938) Report of the chief medical officer: on the state of the public health. HMSO, London

Ministry of Health (1946) Report of the chief medical officer: on the state of the public health. HMSO, London

Ministry of Health (1965a) Medical arrangements for long-stay immigrants. Letter of 4th January 1965 to medical officers of health

Ministry of Health (1965b) Medical arrangements for long-stay immigrants. Letter of 4th January 1965 to general medical practitioners

Ministry of Health (1968) The administrative structure of the medical and related services in England and Wales. HMSO, London

Ministry of Health and Department of Health for Scotland (1944) Venereal disease: guide for practitioners, by Dr LW Harrison

Moir ARM (1962) Annual report of the medical officer of health of Stockport for 1962. Stockport Borough Council, Stockport, Cheshire

Mullan F (1989) Plagues and politics. Basic Books, Inc., New York

Musto DF (1991) Popular and public health responses to tuberculosis in America after 1870. In: Harden VA, Risse GB (eds) Aids and the Historian. US Department of Health and Human Services, Washington, DC

Nabel GJ, Wei C-J, Ledgerwood JE (2011) Vaccinate for the next H2N2 pandemic now. Nature 47:157–158 (Published online 9 March 2011)

National Association for the Promotion of Social Science (1869) Quoted in Lambert R (1963) Sir John Simon 1816–1904. Macgibbon and Kee, London

Newman Sir G (1933) The rise of preventive medicine. Oxford University Press, London

Noah N (2006) Controlling communicable disease. Open University Press, Maidenhead/New York

Nutton V (1983) The seeds of disease—an explanation of contagion from the Greeks to the Renaissance. Med Hist 27(1): 1–34

Nutton V (1990) The reception of Fracastoro's theory of contagion. The seed that fell among thorns. Osiris 2nd series, vol 6. University of Chicago Press, Chicago

O'Mahony M, Stanwell-Smith RE, Tillett HE, Harper D, Hutchison JG, Farrell ID, Hutchinson DN, Lee JV, Dennis PJ and Duggal HV et al (1990) The Stafford outbreak of Legionnaires' disease. Epidemiol Infect 104(3):361–380

Offit PA (2011) Deadly choices: how the anti-vaccine movement threatens as all. Basic Books, New York

Ogunmekan DA (1996) Immunization and other measures for the eradication of listed diseases in Africa. In: Sofoluwe GO, Schram R, Ogunmekan DA (eds) Principles and practice of public health in Africa. University Press PLC, Ibadan

Oriel JD (1994) The scars of Venus: history of venereology. Springer, Berlin/Heidelberg

Pappas G, Ismene JK, Falagas ME (2008) Insights into infectious disease in the era of Hippocrates. Int J Infect Dis 12(4):347–350

Pareek M et al (2011) Screening of immigrants in the UK for imported latent tuberculosis: a multicentre cohort study and cost-effectiveness analysis. Lancet 11(6):435–444 (www.thelancet.com/infection)

Parish HJ (1965) A history of immunization. E&S Livingstone Ltd, Edinburgh

Peckham C, Bedford H, Seenturia Y et al (1989) National immunisation study: factors affecting immunisation in childhood. Action Research for the Crippled Child, Horsham

Pelling M (1978) Cholera, fever and English medicine 1825–1865. Oxford University Press, Oxford

Pennington H (2002) Smallpox scares. London Review of Books 24(17), 5 Sept 2002

Pollock GT (1964) Infective hepatitis in a junior training centre. The Medical Officer 111(21): 301–302

Pollock GT (1984) L'Intégration des médecins à l'administration des services de santé. Proceedings of the 6th Jean-Yves Rivard Colloquium. L'Université de Montréal, Montréal

Pollock GT (1988) "Consensus Management"—peut-il exister dans le National Health Service de l'Angleterre? In: Proceedings of the 4th conference of the international society for system science in health care. L'Université de Lyon, Lyon

Pollock G (1989) Coventry's public health: annual report of the director of public health. Department of Community Medicine, Coventry Health Authority, Coventry

Pollock G (1993) Making London better and communicable disease control. Consultancy Report to the (then) four Thames Regional Health Authorities

Pollock GT, Clayton TM (1964) Epidemic collapse: a mysterious outbreak in three Coventry schools. BMJ 2(5425):1625–1627

Pollock GT, Bhopal R, Duckworth G, McEvoy M, O'Brien S, O'Mahony M, Strangeways J (1994) Training for the CCDC role. Faculty of Public Health Medicine, London

Porter D (1997) Public health and centralisation: the Victorian British state. In: Detels R, Holland WW, McEwen J, Omenn GS (eds) Oxford textbook of public health, 3rd edn. Oxford University Press, Oxford

Porter D (1999) Health, civilization and the state. Routledge, London/New York

Qualtière LF, Slights WWE (2003) Contagion and blame in early Modern England: the case of the French Pox. Lit Med 22(1):1–24

Richardson IM (1956) Introductory lecture, University of Aberdeen 1956/1957 Diploma in Public Health course. 12 October 1956

Rosen G (1958) A history of public health. Johns Hopkins University Press, Baltimore/London

Rymer T (1712) Foedera, v 655. Quoted in Creighton C (1894) A history of epidemics in Britain. Cambridge University Press, Cambridge

Salisbury D, Ramsay M, Noakes K (2006) Immunisation against infectious disease. Department of Health, London

Saunders P (2011) The experience of the 2009–2010 swine flu (H1N1) pandemic in Sandwell. (Internal report, unpublished). Sandwell Primary Health Care Trust, Sandwell

Siena KP (1998) Pollution, promiscuity, and the pox: English venereology and the early modern discourse on social and sexual danger. J Hist Sexuality 8(4):553–574, Published by the University of Chicago

Simon Sir J (1850) General pathology, as conducive to the establishment of rational principles for the diagnosis and treatment of disease. A course of lectures delivered at St Thomas's Hospital, London during the summer of 1850

Smith WH (1873) Smith's family physician. John Lovell, Montreal

Smith F (1945) Coventry: six hundred years of municipal life. Coventry Cathedral Chronicle in association with the Coventry Evening Telegraph, Coventry

Smith FB (1979) The people's health 1830–1910. Croom Helm, London

Snow J (1849) On the mode of communication of cholera. John Churchill, Soho, London

Snow J (1855) On the mode of communication of cholera. Second report. John Churchill, Soho, London

Stern BJ (1927) Should we be vaccinated? Harper and Bros, New York/London

Summers J (1989) Soho—a history of London's most colourful neighbourhood. Bloomsbury, London

The Herald (1897) Obituary of Dr Mark Antony Fenton 9th April 1897. Printed at Earl Street and Palace Yard, Coventry

Tomlinson J (1849) Cholera: special form of prayer to be used during the prevalence of cholera in the country. Printed and sold to be used on Sunday 16 September 1849 by Joseph Tomlinson, High Street, Coventry

Turnbull HM, McIntosh J (1926) Post-vaccinial encephalomyelitis. Br J Exp Pathol 7:81

Vaid N (2010) Private sector providers in England: the implications of Independent Sector Treatment Centres. Eurohealth 16(3):8–10

Wakefield AJ, Murch SH, Anthony A, Linnell J, Casson DM, Malik M et al (1998) Ileal-lymphoid-nodular hyperplasia, non-specific colitis, and pervasive developmental disorder in children. Lancet 351:637–641

Waksman SA (1952) Streptomycin: background, isolation, properties and utilization. Nobel Lecture 12 December 1952

Watson R (2011) MEPs criticise WHO for alarm created by H1N1 pandemic advice. BMJ 342:d652

Watson JM, Pebody RG (2011) Pandemic influenza vaccines. BMJ Editorial 26th February 2011

Watts G (2006) Communicating with patients on the risks and benefits of pharmaceuticals. Eurohealth 12(1):15–16

Welshman J (2000) Municipal medicine: public health in twentieth century Britain. Peter Lang AG, Oxford/Berne

Wenhui L, Swee-Kee W, Fang L et al (2006) Animal origins of the SARS coronavirus: insight from ACE2-S-protein interaction. J Virol (Washington, DC) 80(9):4211–4219

Willan R (1821) Quoted in miscellaneous works of the late Robert Willan. (Ashby Smith Ed.) T Cadell, London

Williams REO (1985) Microbiology for the public health. Public Health Laboratory Service, London

Williams Sir R (1987) The history of the public health laboratory service. In: Farrow S (ed) The public health challenge. Hutchinson, London

Wilson GS (1951) The public health laboratory service. Br Med Bull 7(3):147–153

Wilson GS (1967) The hazards of immunization. Athlone Press, London

World Health Organisation (2003a) Coronavirus never before seen in humans is the cause of SARS. 16 April 2003. WHO, Geneva

World Health Organisation (2003b) WHO recommends new measures to prevent travel-related spread of SARS. 27 March 2003. WHO, Geneva

Index

G. Pollock (ed), *An Epidemiological Odyssey: The Evolution of Communicable Disease Control*, DOI 10.1007/978-94-007-3998-7,

MIX
Papier aus verantwortungsvollen Quellen
Paper from responsible sources
FSC® C105338

If you have any concerns about our products,
you can contact us on
ProductSafety@springernature.com

In case Publisher is established outside the EU,
the EU authorized representative is:
Springer Nature Customer Service Center GmbH
Europaplatz 3, 69115 Heidelberg, Germany

Printed by Libri Plureos GmbH
in Hamburg, Germany